"Anyone who looks after older persons knows that end-stage dementia is no different than terminal cancer. The patient requires humane care, needs protection from the juggernaut of modern medicine, and above all deserves a medical team who will deal with symptoms first. Finally, we have a book that deals head-on with this important public health issue. In his usual clear and direct manner, Michael Gordon, a world-renowned geriatrician, and his associate Natalie Baker handle this issue with aplomb. Health care workers, family members of those suffering from dementia, and policymakers all would do very well to read this book and take in its critically important message."

A. Mark Clarfield, MD, FRCPC
Sidonie Hecht Professor of Geriatrics
Ben-Gurion University of the Negev

"Dr. Gordon's work shines light on the special needs of individuals living in the late stage of dementia. A chief priority for all carers is to treat every individual with dementia with respect and dignity throughout the course of the disease. This book provides empathic, practical advice to help with the unique challenges that come with care in the later stages of dementia."

Mary E. Schulz
Director, Information, Support Services, and Education
Alzheimer Society of Canada

"Michael Gordon has written what might be called another 'guide for the perplexed.' In our time, the perplexed are professional and family caregivers of people diagnosed with dementia. Herein he provides a sensitive, insightful, nuanced, and deep understanding of fundamental issues, and supports the dignity and well-being of all concerned. Dr. Gordon is truly a healer whose experience as a geriatrician provides a road map for all of us who want to provide care, respect, and love for people diagnosed with dementia."

Steven R. Sabat, PhD
Professor, Department of Psychology
Georgetown University

"This guide provides a thoughtful narrative review of late-stage dementia with the inclusion of clinical commentary from a well-respected, expert clinician. Particularly helpful is the overview of issues around advanced care planning which is useful for clinicians, patients, and their family members."

Sharon Straus, MD, FRCPC
Professor of Medicine and Geriatrics
University of Toronto

"Essential reading for families of patients with dementia. They will find this book invaluable."

Professor Marion E. T. McMurdo
Head of Ageing and Health
Ninewells Hospital and Medical School
University of Dundee

"From Dr. Gordon's book, families will learn much about helping patients with dementia, but so too will physicians and other caregivers. Michael Gordon's humanity shines through every page and, when combined with his medical expertise, the result is a guide which is both truly thoughtful and practically useful."

Professor Arthur Schafer
Director, Centre for Professional and Applied Ethics
University of Manitoba

"Dr. Gordon has produced a valuable resource for families and friends of loved ones suffering from late-stage dementia and the health care providers who care for these patients. Filled with sage advice from decades of experience, he provides essential information to help loved ones to engage in needed discussions about preferences for care at the end of life by 'having the conversation' as well as to make difficult decisions about care. Included is a helpful guide for clinicians about managing the many clinical problems that inevitably arise."

Arlene S. Bierman, MD, MS
OWHC Chair in Women's Health
University of Toronto

"This is an extremely well-considered guide, in which Dr. Gordon addresses the most challenging issues in late-stage dementia with intelligence, a wealth of experience, and compassion. It provides essential guidance for families and health care professionals caring for patients with end-stage dementia that is ethically based and clinically sound."

Susan L. Mitchell, MD, MPH
Associate Professor of Medicine, Harvard Medical School
Senior Scientist, Hebrew Senior Life Institute for Aging Research

"This book should be required reading for anyone working in this field. I cannot recommend it highly enough."

Laura Watts
National Director
Canadian Centre for Elder Law

"Dr. Gordon brings us his rich experience in medicine and ethics, clear analysis, and understanding of the real dilemmas faced by patients and their caregivers. The result is an important guide that is both instructive and warmly engaging."

Peter R. Newman, MD
Department of Family and Community Medicine
University of Toronto

"I would highly recommend this book to families and health professionals. Dr. Gordon deals with the difficult issues of end-of-life care in those with dementia with practical suggestions and strategies. This book is like having your own personal geriatrician assist with end-of-life dementia care."

Dr. Alexandra Papaioannou
MD, MSc, FRCPC, FACP
Geriatrician Hamilton Health Sciences
Professor of Medicine—Division of Geriatrics
McMaster University

Contents

Acknowledgements   xiii

PART ONE   1

Introduction   3
Why this guide?   3
Dementia: A Brief Overview   4
Consider the Case of Mary   5
Dr. Gordon Discusses   6
Dementia: Denial and Disbelief   7
Dementia: A Terminal Disease?   9
Dr. Gordon Discusses   11
Summary   12

Why Palliative Care?   14
The Clinical Course of Dementia   14
Dr. Gordon Discusses   15
Defining Palliative Care   15
Dr. Gordon Discusses   18
Summary   20

PART TWO   23

Decision-Making and Ethical Decisions   25
Advanced Care Planning   25
An Ethical Approach   25
Communication   27
Dr. Gordon Discusses   27
Informed Consent   28
Information Disclosure   29
Capacity   29
Substitute Decision-making   30
Discussing Patient History   32

Decision-Making   32
Dr. Gordon Discusses   32
Confidentiality, Privacy, and Respectfulness   34
Nutrition and Hydration   35
Dr. Gordon Discusses   37
Pain and Other Symptoms   39
Withholding or Stopping Life-Sustaining Treatments   40
Dealing with Conflict   41
Summary   42

PART THREE   **43**

Comfort Care in Context   45
End of Life through Different Cultural Lenses   45
Dr. Gordon Discusses   46
Cultural Influence   47
Summary   48

Caring for the Caregiver   49
Emotional Distress   49
Dr. Gordon Discusses   50
The Process of Caregiving   51
Loss and Grief   52
Dr. Gordon Discusses   53
Transcendence: Different Ways of Connecting   54
Coping with Grief   55
Summary   56

A Sense of Autonomy   57
Taking the Perspective of the Patient   57
Dr. Gordon Discusses   59
A Call for Education   60
Summary   61

Avoiding and Dealing with Family Conflict   62
Despite Best Efforts   62
Dr. Gordon Discusses   64
Summary   65

Appendix A: Symptom Management: Maintaining Comfort   67

   Managing Symptoms   67
   Assessing Symptoms   68

Symptom   71

   Depression   71
   Anxiety   75
   Weight Loss/Anorexia/Cachexia   77
   Constipation   81
   Nausea/Vomiting   88
   Delirium   91
   Dyspnea/Breathlessness/Respiratory Problems   94
   Dysphagia/Oral Complications   97
   Skin Breakdown/Chronic Wounds   102
   Dehydration   108
   Pain   110

Appendix B: Useful Scales, Assesment Tools, and
Medications for Symptom Management   119

Glossary of Commonly Used Ethical Terms   143

References and Further Reading   149

Resources   153

Index   155

Acknowledgements

A great deal of work and support went into the production of this guide. From the time of the initial proposal to the Innovation Fund organized by the Ontario Ministry of Health and Long-Term Care, I received encouragement in support from the Alzheimer Society of Canada through its office in Toronto. To the staff in that office, I am indebted for their faith in me. During the development of the concepts that became the foundation of the guide, the help of Dr. Daphna Grossman of the Palliative Care Program at Baycrest Geriatric Health Care System and Dr. Marcia Sokolowski, ethicist at Baycrest, were very helpful and supportive in the evolution of the guide. I also wish to thank Leslie Iancovitz, Julie Grossman, Mary McDiarmid, and Anne Kirstein of Baycrest; Mary Schulz, Debbie Benczkowski, and Scott Dudgeon of the Alzheimer Society of Canada; Dr. Lawrence Librach of the Temmy Latner Centre for Palliative Care, Toronto; Professor Steven Sabat of Georgetown University; Dr. Susan Mitchell of Harvard University; and Trish Staples for the time and effort that they took to read the manuscript and make suggestions for its improvement. I especially wish to thank Steve Cowan from the Baycrest print shop for assisting in preparing the poster used to present the guide at the Innovation Fund Showcase, as well as the draft copies of the formatted manuscript.

I want to particularly thank Natalie Baker, the project manager of this guide, who undertook to read everything imaginable on the subject and who collated all the information and molded it into the manuscript that became the basis of the guide. She was an endless source of inspiration and good humor as she brought together all the information into a cohesive form and interwove my personal anecdotes into the content of the text.

I am indebted to the authors of the Baycrest Palliative Care Manual, who years ago created this resource for the physicians who work at Baycrest and are confronted with medication and other care challenges of those admitted to the palliative care program. The primary author of that manual is Daniel Buchman, who was a pleasure to work with, both on that and on other summer projects that he undertook while still a student. I also want to thank the editors and staff of the *Canadian Jewish News* for allowing me to write a monthly column, "The Senior Side of Life," directed to seniors and their families, from which many excerpts are used in this guide.

Lastly, I want to thank the many patients and families I have worked with over the years for being the source of my continual inspiration, motivation, and passion to help them achieve their goals.

PART ONE

INTRODUCTION

Why this guide?

Many highly industrialized countries face a rapidly aging population. According to Statistics Canada, one in eight Canadians in 2001 was aged 65 years or over, and by 2026, one Canadian in five will have reached age 65. It is imperative then that age-related illness and end-of-life care are more closely and openly discussed and understood among health care professionals and in the public forum.

In recent years, there has been an increased knowledge and awareness of Alzheimer's disease and other causes of dementia by health care professionals and the general public. This is in part thanks to the efforts of organizations, such as the Alzheimer Society of Canada and the Alzheimer Association in the United States, that are committed to addressing the challenges associated with the care of those living with dementia. This is also due to the development and marketing of medications that can ameliorate symptoms and affect the course of diseases that cause dementia. Even if these initiatives have been motivated partially by the pharmaceutical industry's financial interests, ultimately it has meant that it is now part of the normal discourse to identify individuals with cognitive impairment and to focus on interventions that might be of value.

At first it may sound a bit counterintuitive to frame the more recent spotlight on end-of-life issues in a positive light. However, an aging population and the accompanying abundance of age-related issues translates into the reality that many more people are living longer than ever before. There was a time when there wasn't a significant need for discussions regarding end-of-life issues or for guidelines for caregivers and health care professionals. This is because, in the past, individuals would have a much steeper end-of-life trajectory after falling ill in old age. Now, thanks to significant medical advances, there is an average length of four and a half years spent by patients in a long-term care home before they die. Many older people die at home after long and disabling illnesses. In order to remain at home during this last period of life, there is often the need for help from family members, friends, neighbors, and home care services. Accordingly, this means that there are new end-of-life challenges and procedures that must be discussed, debated, and hopefully resolved. This is the starting point of this guide.

Dementia: A Brief Overview

Dementia is a general term that is used to describe a condition that affects primarily older individuals whose memory, judgment, and other cognitive functions decline; frequently this is accompanied by abnormal behavior, such as agitation and suspiciousness. Dementia has many causes and thus many variations in both the way symptoms occur and in the impact on cognitive function and emotional state.

Alzheimer's disease *is the leading form of dementia*. It currently represents 63 percent of all dementias. What is known as vascular, or multi-infarct, dementia accounts for about 20 percent of all cases. Both forms are caused by the death of cells, which, in the case of the vascular component of the disease, is due to blockages of the many small blood vessels in the brain. This results in the brain cells being deprived of oxygen and essential nutrients. Both types of dementia can occur in isolation or in combination—a common occurrence, particularly for those who are getting on in their years.

Much of the effort during the past few years has been on understanding the mechanisms of disease that cause the different kinds of dementia and on what might be done to decrease the risk and possibly treat the various symptoms. We have come to recognize that although there are likely different categories of dementia, there is a good deal of overlap between the various types of dementia that affect most individuals.

There is an overlap both in terms of the risk factors and the usual steps suggested in order to mitigate these risk factors. Many of these steps are lifestyle related and include: the cessation of smoking, regular exercise, and proper diet, plus the control of hypertension (high blood pressure), hyper-lipidemia (elevated or abnormal blood fats), and diabetes mellitus.

For other less common causes of dementia, there are some interventions that may be useful in specific cases, but for the vast majority of those who experience a dementia-causing illness, the approach noted above is fairly consistent. In addition, many researchers and scientists argue that there are other steps that individuals can take to decrease the risk of the disease or perhaps slow the progression of it. These may include challenging brain function through brain exercises such as crossword puzzles and brain teasers, as well as avoiding head injury, for example from sports accidents. Whether the use of psychoactive substances such as recreational drugs may play a role is not clear, but most physicians would cautiously suggest that individuals avoid the use of substances for this and other health care-related reasons. For example, alcohol abuse has long been known to cause injury to the brain, and prolonged use can result in dementia. In those with the propensity to other types of dementia, alcohol can be an additive factor in its causation.

Physicians typically use a control or curative model when dealing with many illnesses, and this tends to be the same when approaching patients with dementia. Even though there is no cure for dementia at any stage, the general medical approach is to use those available, proven medications to ease the symptoms as the disease progresses. The goal is to diagnose and treat the dementia as early and effectively as possible and to maintain as much function as possible for as long as possible.

During the past decade, a number of medications have been introduced that purportedly improve some aspects of function in those living with dementia, as well as perhaps decrease the rate of clinical decline. Although there has been some controversy as to the efficacy of these medications in North America, they are widely used, both alone and in combination. Additionally, it is sometimes necessary to use behaviour-modifying medications when dementia-related behaviours do not respond to behavioural modifications, environmental interventions, and various other non-pharmacological interventions. These include antidepressants and various minor and major tranquilizers, often in the class called *neuroleptics*, including a newer variety called the *atypical neuroleptics*.

Consider the Case of Mary

(This is a fictionalized synthesis of a number of real cases that share common themes with the emphasis on one case in which the sex, name, and other details of the case have been altered to respect the privacy of the individuals involved in the story.)

Mary was an eighty-eight-year-old woman admitted to complex continuing care from an adjacent long-term care facility for a pulmonary tract (lung) infection. She lived with dementia and had gradually declined in function during the preceding four years, having lived for three years in the retirement home. The aspiration pneumonia was not the first episode of pneumonia she had during the preceding year, and her attending physician was aware of her declining function and general disability. She had difficulty recognizing people and was even at times prone to mixing up close members of her family. In terms of basic *activities of daily living* (ADLs), Mary needed help in all aspects of care. For example, she often kept food in her mouth for long periods of time before either swallowing or spitting it out, and was by this time doubly incontinent; that is, she could not control her bowel movements or her urination.

The family, distraught by her decline, continued to search for treatments that might improve her cognition and decrease her risk of infection. The focus was essentially on keeping their mother alive. Though never actually having had this particular conversation with her, they had rejected in principle any thought of artificial nutrition and hydration, as they believed that is not what she would have wanted. End-of-life preferences in general were never discussed when she might have been able to engage in such matters; her family felt that this kind of conversation would have been too painfully upsetting for their mother.

After a recovery from the aspiration pneumonia, Mary experienced another similar episode, and the attending physician asked the family what they would like to do. Searching for guidance, they asked the physician for options, and she outlined various interventions, including some imaging studies and blood work that might help "diagnose" the problem. The physician, however, did not bring up the option of end-of-life care, in keeping with a palliative approach to current and future care. A short time later, the patient passed away after another course of antibiotics and some limited symptomatic treatment to address difficulty breathing and severe shortness of breath with associated agitation. The physician explained that she was reluctant to use morphine, other than in very small doses, for example, to decrease the respiratory symptoms. She explained that she "could not do anything that would seemingly be responsible for ending the patient's life prematurely."

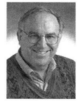

Dr. Gordon Discusses

Note to readers: In this book when the issue is part of the "Dr. Gordon Discusses" section, the text will be italicized to highlight this more

personalized portion of the book and to separate it from the other sections.

It is clear from the fictionalized anecdote that Mary's physician did all that she could do to respond to the wishes of Mary's family and prolong their mother's life. In fact, this is exactly the issue that needs to be examined: in essence, **Mary's quantity of life was favoured over her quality of life.** *While this is certainly understandable from a cultural, religious, or even a simply emotional perspective (families often have an instinctive desire to keep their loved ones alive for as long as possible), there are many detrimental effects of taking solely this curative, interventional approach to end-stage dementia.*

Dementia: Denial and Disbelief

First of all, the effectiveness of using an aggressive medical approach in dealing with end-stage dementia must be questioned when patients often must endure high levels of discomfort for a relatively low return.

There are objective ways of defining what is meant by end-stage dementia. One of the evaluation scales is called the Global Deterioration Scale and is used by clinicians and researchers worldwide to measure the level of function of those living with dementia. It is also a good indicator of the expected trajectory for future life. The clinical picture as the end of life is approaching usually consists of a vocabulary that has become very limited, and then verbal abilities eventually disappear. There is usually a loss of ability to walk independently and sit without support. There is also the need for help with eating and using the toilet. Most people in this stage of progression are usually incontinent.

By the end stages of dementia, the process of decline can be generally predicted, and even though an exact prognosis may not be defined, the general time period is rarely as long as six months and is more likely anywhere from one to six months. Evidence has shown that end-stage dementia is associated with a poor prognosis, and invasive treatments do not significantly improve the duration of life. Thus the downside of these medical advances may result in the unrealistic priority to sustain or lengthen life. This may paradoxically lead to further suffering due to ineffectual medical procedures and treatments.

Additionally, there now is such a great focus on medical treatments that conversations and decision-making about the dying process may seem to be even harder to initiate than ever before. In previous generations, death was put not in a medical or hospital context, but in a social, cultural, or religious context, and this helped to give the dying process meaning for the terminally ill person and his or her family. Equally challenging are religious perspectives that support all measures that promote life, even under very trying and challenging circumstances. Physicians and other health care professionals must be aware of the impact of such belief systems on the decision-making that goes into end-of-life care. Sometimes religious consultants might be of assistance to families who need to both find ways to accept the reality of the end-of-life situation and also make decisions on behalf of their loved one.

There has been a kind of "medicalization" of death in contemporary society, creating almost a universal conspiracy of silence surrounding the process of death and dying. There is often a lack of communication when it comes to discussions about the natural course of diseases causing dementia and the terminal stage of the disorder. This is the time (ideally early on in the disease trajectory) where important planning and decisions about end-of-life care should be part of the dialogue between patients, their families, and physicians responsible for care. The result of this silence is often a series of aggressive medical interventions and then shock and/or denial when the terminal stages of dementia do occur. There is typically little preparation or communication about how to approach the care needs at this point.

For most people and their families who are confronted with a diagnosis of dementia, the initial response is often a combination of denial and disbelief, as well as a quest for potentially reversible causes or aggravating factors. Some patients and families go from one physician to another trying to determine whether or not the diagnosis is "certain." Often the patient gains little insight or understanding of the condition. This can lead to many problems, as the person is not aware of the deficiencies in cognition and function and may be very upset as steps are taken, for example, to assure their safety as well as the safety of others. This point is often dramatically brought home to families when it becomes necessary to report the diagnosis of dementia to the motor vehicle bureau, usually resulting in a loss of one's driver's license. This may cause a terrible loss of both self-esteem and sense of independence in the person living with dementia. The decision often causes strife in the family, as the patient may not understand why the step has been taken and may accuse the family of being responsible for it, especially when the medical appointment was arranged by the family in the first place.

One of the problems that family members face is the sense that *the process has no end*. There usually is a very slow, progressive decline in function, with the family members undertaking all kinds of steps to increase care and attention so that life can go on. For much of this process, the person suffering from dementia can participate in many activities of life and find enjoyment in some aspects of life and relationships. This might normally be the time to discuss the long-term prognosis and expected outcome. As this period of the disease may last some years, discussion about treatment and care preferences for later on may not occur. These discussions best take place while the person affected by the disease still has the cognitive abilities to tell others of their wishes.

A common question often raised by family members is, "When is the right time or best time to discuss end-of-life decisions or preferences?" In some ways, the optimal time is when there is nothing wrong with the person so that the discussion is dispassionate and almost theoretical, as if one were talking about a third person, even though it is meant to be personalized. It might be asked as, "What would you prefer to have done should you be in the following state of function?" Sometimes it is hard for a person to imagine such a state, but many times there has been a situation with another family member or friend. If this situation can be referred to as an example, it might become clear to the person that what was done to that other person represents a state or decision that they would either accept or reject.

Dementia: A Terminal Disease?

We have suggested that the so-called "medicalization of death" has contributed to some of the silence surrounding end-stage dementia decision-making. The upside of these medical advances is that they can also offer opportunities to improve the end-stage dementia process. There is the option of taking a *palliative care approach,* which places the alleviation of pain, other clinical symptoms, and suffering as the main objective of care. While this is a quite widely known and accepted approach in terminal cancers, for example, it has yet to reach the same widespread usage and acceptance in terms of applying it to Alzheimer's disease and related dementias. Part of the reason is that dementia is not typically conceptualized as a terminal illness.

Whereas other terminal illnesses can take a relatively quick, predictable decline, the trajectory of a patient with dementia can be slow and variable. These time and speed factors may account for some of the denial around issues of death, the hesitancy to label dementia as a terminal illness, and the lack of communication surrounding treatments that may be most suitable for the end stage of illness. This silence, and the barriers it creates, means that physicians don't yet have the confidence or assurance to implement some of the palliative care approaches and treatments on patients. For example, the effective administration of narcotics may be appropriate in order to help reduce suffering.

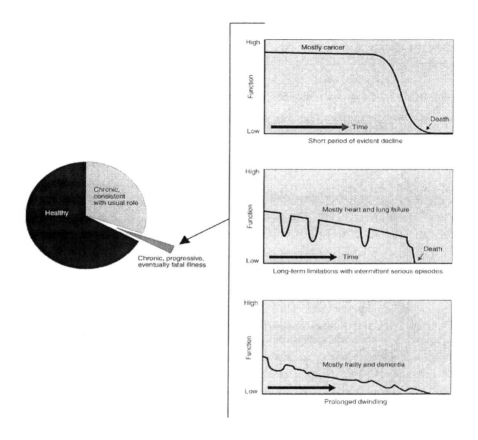

Adapted from: Lynn J, Adamson DM, *Living well at the end-of-life. Adapting health care to serious chronic illness in old age. Washington: Rand Health, 2003.*

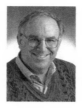

Dr. Gordon Discusses

During most of my forty years of medical practice, the concept of terminal disease seemed to be reasonably clear. Recently, a fellow Baycrest hospital staff member said to me, "I have never heard of Alzheimer's disease being categorized as a terminal disease. Cancer I know is often spoken about in that fashion, but how can the same be said for Alzheimer's disease?" The question was an important one: without an understanding of the course of this devastating disease, patients may not receive the appropriate and necessary care and may not be provided with the proper information needed to make autonomous current and future medical decisions. The usual conceptual framework and terminology that we use for "terminal disease" is flawed. These flaws affect our approach to those we treat, how we communicate, how public policy is formulated, and how health care is delivered, essentially impacting the ethical principle of resource allocation.

Historically, health care professionals characterized a terminal disease as one for which there was little effective treatment and the trajectory or death from the time of diagnosis until the end was relatively short and fairly predictable. Traditionally the prototypical terminal disease was cancer. I can recall years ago that it was common to think of the person as having a "terminal disease" even before the "terminal" phase of its course.

One of the great achievements of modern medicine is the transformation of many previously untreatable diseases into what is now conceptualized as chronic disease—conditions that can be controlled for years or decades with good function and close to normal life activities, as long as the necessary treatment regimens are followed. Rather than thinking of diseases as terminal or not, it seems preferable to think of all diseases as having a course that at some point, may enter a terminal phase.

For example, Alzheimer's disease starts with a perhaps five- or ten-year long preclinical state, characterized by a gradual loss and change of critical cells in certain parts of the brain, such as the hippocampus. As the microscopic tell-tale tangles and plaques develop further, the person demonstrates the clinically recognized cognitive and personality changes. Over the next number of years, despite current pharmacologic treatments, there is progression with further cognitive and behavioral change.

This is when families struggle with issues related to function and whether relative independence can be maintained. This is the stage of decline, but not the terminal stage, of the disease. Over time patients incrementally lose their ability to do basic activities of daily living and eventually some critical activities, including the ability to eat and drink. With swallowing problems comes an increased risk for inflammation and irritation of the lungs from inhaled food and fluids (aspiration pneumonia) and also a decline in the immune system as it becomes more and more difficult to maintain a healthy and sufficient diet.

In the preterminal state of the disease, patients become increasingly immobile, bed-bound, and totally dependent. At this point, the critical steps leading to the terminal phase include raising the question of whether the process of considering future care will address the option of providing parenteral (through one sort of tube or another) feeding. Once repeated infections occur, the person starts down the path to the "terminal" phase of the disease. Ultimately, the same decisions that have to be made in late-stage malignant disease come into play: the limits of care and medical interventions, such as whether or not to treat unrelated illnesses, or as noted above, the use of feeding tubes.

With this construction of the concept of terminal diseases, one could use the terminology "terminal stage of …" cancer, Alzheimer's disease, heart failure, kidney failure, Parkinson's disease, and so on. The importance of communicating the implications of these diseases so that patients can be informed and participate in their own decision-making must be emphasized. If families acting as surrogates or substitute decision-makers have already accepted that their loved one is in the terminal phase of a long-standing disease, the later decisions might be easier to prepare for and make.

Summary

We want this guide to be a part of the growing number of resources that contribute to the knowledge dissemination process amongst professionals and caregivers working with patients living with end-stage dementia. We believe that education and awareness are necessary in order to break the silence around issues of end-stage dementia and more generally about the process of dying itself. We have put together a set of topics and guidelines that are intended for professionals in this field, patients with dementia, and their families and/or caregivers.

Our hope is that these kinds of initiatives will lead to greater knowledge and understanding, and ultimately to widespread progress in treatment and care approaches.

It is critical in developing an approach to care to remember that:

- All the various causes of dementia result in a progressive disease, a disease where function continues to decline over time. Interventions cannot restore function, merely slow down the decline and ease the symptoms.
- In the latter stages of dementia, critical self-care and protective capabilities of the person living with dementia decline and the person becomes increasingly dependent on others for basic care.
- Eventually people living with dementia enter a preterminal and then terminal stage of their disease, where they are susceptible to infections and accidental falls, which often lead to death.
- It is important for family members and clinicians to recognize and accept that, when dementia is clearly in its terminal phase, the focus of care should be on symptom relief rather than acute medical interventions that rarely provide benefit and often result in prolonging suffering.
- At some point in the process, the issue of artificial feeding will likely have to be addressed. It is important that those involved in the decision-making process understand the benefits and risks of such an intervention and the basis on which such a profound decision is generally made (see Part Two: Nutrition and Hydration and Dr. Gordon Discusses Feeding Tubes).

WHY PALLIATIVE CARE?

The Clinical Course of Dementia

> Dementia is a terminal illness and needs to be recognized
> as such so these patients receive better palliative care.
>
> —Dr. Susan L. Mitchell (Professor of Geriatric
> Medicine, Harvard University, 2009)

There is a lack of understanding about the physical toll of dementia and the typical trajectory that this disease takes. A recently published paper by a group of Harvard researchers addressed this issue by conducting a prospective, observational study of 323 patients with advanced dementia in 22 nursing homes in the Boston area and followed the patients for up to 18 months (Mitchell et al., 2009). The aim of the study was to provide a better understanding of the clinical epidemiology and lifespan course of this particular population.

The results showed that most of the participants could not communicate verbally (and the ones who could had a vocabulary of fewer than six words), could not walk independently, were unable to recognize members of their family, and were incontinent. Sadly, nearly a quarter of the participants passed away within six months of enrolling in the study, and by the time the study had concluded, more than half of the dementia patients had passed away. These patients died as a result of their dementia. L. Volicer from the University of South Florida, in a 2005 literature review from the Alzheimer's Association, showed similar trends in end-of-life care. That the exact cause of death was due to conditions related to their underlying dementia, such as eating problems or infections, is not as important as understanding that it was the dementia that was the "cause" of their death.

The literature indicates that given these distressing symptoms and this overall prognosis, it is helpful to view advanced dementia as a terminal illness so that patients can avoid being subjected to painful medical interventions and be given the option of palliative care instead. It is important to take note that the perceptions of the patients' caregivers determined whether or not a palliative approach was taken. More specifically, according to Mitchell et al. (2009), if the proxy perceived that their loved one had six months or fewer to live and understood the high likelihood for medical complications, they were far less likely to initiate complex medical interventions for the patient.

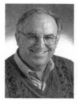

Dr. Gordon Discusses

I believe that the biggest challenge in this field is for physicians and nurses to understand and help educate their patients and/or families about the natural outcome of dementia. It is a condition with a gradual decline that includes the loss of many important attributes, including the ability to feed oneself or to respond to interactions and stimulations. The person becomes prone to co-morbidities, including infection and other conditions that are pervasive in the older population. Clinicians must be prepared to provide all the potentially effective clinical treatments to provide symptomatic care combined with robust emotionally supportive care. They should not get caught up in searching for things that can be "treated," even for a short time, while neglecting to address the true suffering that patients and their families experience during this time.

Defining Palliative Care

What exactly is meant by the term "palliative care"? Essentially, palliative care is the term used to describe care that is not curative in nature, where the goal is to prevent and relieve suffering, and to support the best quality of life for patients and their families. While palliative care is usually thought of as care provided in the terminal stages of a disease—care when there is no hope of cure—in reality, patients receive enormous benefit from palliative care regardless of the stage of their disease. It is increasingly more common to refer to the subset of palliative care provided at the end of life as just that: end-of-life care. The components of palliative care include addressing physical symptoms that cause any kind of discomfort, such as pain, nausea, and difficulty breathing. It is also no less important to address the psychosocial and spiritual aspects of caring in order to achieve a modicum of serenity as life is coming to an end.

The Canadian Palliative Care Association further clarifies palliative care as:

- A special kind of health care for individuals and families who are living with a life-threatening illness that is usually at an advanced stage.
- The goal of palliative care is comfort and dignity for the person living with the illness as well as the best quality of life for both this person and his or her family.
- A 'family' is whoever the person says his or her family is. It may include relatives, partners, and friends.
- An important objective of palliative care is relief of pain and other symptoms.
- Palliative care is planned to meet not only physical needs but also the psychological, social, cultural, emotional, and spiritual needs of each person and family.
- Palliative care may be the main focus of care when a cure for the illness is no longer possible. Palliative care services help people in later life who are ill to live out their remaining time in comfort and dignity.

One could argue that, in fact, the principles of palliative care should be part of all medical interactions in terms of the focus on the individual and the quality of life. The main difference in common clinical practice is that when a "cure" or a major change in the trajectory of illness is being sought, the subtler aspects and nuances of quality of care and sensitivity to the individual may be overlooked or forgotten in the urgency and complexity of life-maintaining or life-saving medical interventions.

In the field of cancer care, when palliative care is discussed, it is sometimes combined within a framework of *simultaneous care*. According to a Cancer Care Ontario (CCO) 2009 document, "a simultaneous care approach focuses on helping patients move through the trajectory of a progressive, life-threatening disease by enabling their changing goals of care to be met at all stages based on an interdisciplinary approach to care that attends to symptom management, psychosocial issues, and advance-care planning. A simultaneous approach to care embraces the concept of palliative care being applicable early in the course of the disease, in conjunction with other therapies that are intended to prolong life, such as chemotherapy or radiation therapy. The simultaneous approach supports the definition of "palliative care" being distinguished from that of "end-of-life care," which specifically refers to services provided to dying patients and their families. By embracing a simultaneous approach to care, the CCO Palliative Care Program allows for earlier identification, documentation, and communication of symptoms, thereby decreasing time to optimal symptom management and, if necessary, referral to appropriate members of a multidisciplinary team."

Although this concept works well in those living with cancer, it is somewhat less suitable for those living with dementia. The applicability of simultaneous care to those living with dementia is that early on in the disease trajectory, when symptoms are mild, most individuals welcome and respond to interventions for other health care issues that may respond to treatment without in any way improving the course of dementia but can assure a higher quality of life than might have been expected had their conditions not been addressed. For example, the treatment of heart disease and arthritis or diabetes in older people living with dementia will likely improve their function and quality of life, even if by doing so the trajectory of the progress of the dementia is not substantially altered. In such situations, most physicians, patients, and families would pursue appropriate interventions as long as the result does not aggravate the symptoms of dementia and the functional decline associated with it.

It is important that health care professionals and caregivers conceptualize dementia as a disease with a well-recognized terminal phase; a salient feature of palliative care is the recognition that, during this latter stage of the condition, many relatively minor events can be life-threatening. At some point, because of the loss of resilience due to the underling dementia, death becomes inevitable and imminent. This may be difficult to grasp by family members and other loved ones because the course of the disease can be fairly slow compared to other fatal illnesses. As opposed to a steep downhill course in the last few months, as is the case with an aggressive case of cancer, severe dementia is more likely to go downhill in a slower, somewhat more variable way. This can give caregivers a sense of hope, a sense that things will improve, and that medical interventions will reverse their loved one's condition. Unfortunately there is much evidence that more aggressive interventions such as laboratory tests, restraints in an attempt to prevent devastating falls, or intravenous therapy do not change the course of the dying process. Tube feeding, in general, is ultimately more of a hindrance to the quality of the dying process than a help (Finucane et al., 1999; Mitchell et al., 2009). (See Part Two: Nutrition and Hydration and Dr. Gordon Discusses Feeding Tubes.)

Though it can be hard for caregivers, especially close family members, once they recognize and accept that their loved one's illness is not curable, taking a palliative approach makes things as comfortable and supportive as possible for all those involved.

It should be clarified here that the point of palliative care is not to hasten death or to postpone it. To reiterate: the main purpose of this kind of care is to provide relief from unpleasant symptoms and to incorporate some spiritual and/or psychological aspects of care, including providing support for not only patients with dementia but also their friends and family. If done properly, it is the rare occurrence that proper palliative care and symptom management measures hasten death. Rather, they make the process better tolerated and relieve suffering.

> We're not talking about aggressive care versus no care. Palliative care is aggressive and attentive and focused on symptom management and support of the patient and family. It's not any less excellent care.
>
> —Dr. Greg A. Sachs (Professor of Medicine, Researcher, and Chief of the Division of General Internal Medicine and Geriatrics at Indiana University, 2004)

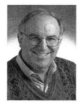

Dr. Gordon Discusses

"You might as well just kill her. Why not shoot her and get it over with?"
"It is an act of euthanasia. I thought euthanasia was outlawed in this country."
"I am going to report you to the media. You can't just kill people, you know."
"Stopping the respirator is the same as killing her. Is that the business you are in?"

These are some of the comments I have heard over the past few years from family members faced with the conundrum of discontinuing life-sustaining respirator treatment. The relatively recent story of Winnipeg Orthodox Jew, Samuel Golubchuk, greatly fueled the flame of controversy. His family chose to keep him on a respirator after his physicians felt that life-support should be discontinued.

For many Orthodox Jews, there is a belief in a religious obligation to maintain life almost at all costs, regardless of the quality of the life that will be sustained. The Canadian and Israeli media weighed in, with some writers characterizing the situation as euthanasia. Some religious leaders took up the mantle as one of religious freedom. Golubchuk passed away prior to the case going to trial. It was described as "natural" by the family, as it was not hastened by the discontinuation of medical life-support systems (Solomon, S., 2008).

How are health care providers who pursue the best life-saving treatments to deal with allegations that, when families believe that the efforts of health care providers have been unsuccessful, these health care providers are accused of being "cruel," "ignoring religious beliefs," or "killing beloved family members"? Physicians who provide life-support and are knowledgeable in the limits of life-support methods can usually accurately predict when recovery is unlikely and thus when further treatment will not be clinically beneficial. This medical perspective may conflict with the family's non-medical, personal, religious, and psychological perspective. Losing a loved one is never easy—having the process interface with the complexities of the modern medical technology does not make it easier.

Prior to the advances in life-support technologies, many older individuals, especially with late-stage heart, brain, and kidney diseases, died from their diseases without any attempt to prolong their life, without any hope that there might be some recovery. Therefore, there was no option of offering life-sustaining treatment. With the increased access and use of life-support technologies, it has become common for individuals with previously fatal diseases to receive a temporary reprieve from death. The rationale is that, on occasion, some individuals recover from the illnesses that previously would have led to their death. With such treatments, some do recover, even if they are left with severe disabilities or unfortunately in permanent coma or some comparable state. The new standard for life-support has become, in essence, "give people the best possible chance for recovery."

The problem occurs when the life-support treatment does not achieve its goal, and then it has to be discontinued. One cannot keep a person on life-support indefinitely. That is the emotional problem for families and for some with strong religious convictions—it is easier to not start a treatment than to stop it. But if we do not agree that if recovery doesn't happen, life-support must be stopped, we could end up depriving people of the chance to respond to such attempts at treatment. Using life-support is not natural as a means of keeping someone alive—it is artificial. Allowing someone to die from their disease after life-support has been tried but failed is natural, and it must be allowed to happen with the tenderness, care, and love that the person deserves, not with the sense of hostility, anger, and disapproval that unfortunately often occurs. Sometimes it is erroneously assumed by families that life-support interventions are without their own measure of discomfort. Many life-support interventions are very uncomfortable for the person, and interventions such as cardiopulmonary resuscitation may result in a person's final experience being one of physical discomfort, as well as the loss of a dignified death. One should not have to pass through the jaws of ineffectual technology to leave this world.

Summary

Palliative care is:

- An approach that **improves the quality of life of patients and families who are facing a life-threatening illness, through the prevention and relief of suffering**. This is achieved through early identification, impeccable assessment, and careful treatment of physical, psychosocial, and spiritual symptoms.

The main goals of palliative care in the end stages of dementia are to:

- Provide relief from pain and other distressing symptoms;
- Affirm life and regard dying as a normal process;
- Intend neither to hasten nor postpone death;
- Integrate the psychological and spiritual aspects of patient care;
- Offer a support system to help patients live as actively as possible until death;
- Offer a support system to help the family cope during the patient's illness and in their own bereavement;
- Use a team approach to address the needs of patients and their families, including bereavement counseling; and
- Enhance quality of life and positively influence the course of the illness.

In order to improve end-of-life care, the following three aspects should be emphasized and will be covered more extensively in the following sections:

1. **Comfort** is a top priority for palliative care in dementia. Pain and other distressing symptoms should be controlled with care and if possible completely alleviated. Nobody should ever have to end their life in suffering. This will enhance the quality of life in the last days of illness.

2. **Decision-making** about life-sustaining treatments and other concerns regarding the patient's last days is well informed. Ideally the decision-making

process should begin early, when the patient is well enough to communicate his or her desires and also to choose a substitute decision-maker for when he or she can no longer decide these issues independently.

3. **Support** is given not only to patients but also to their caregivers. Support may come in many different forms, from recognizing the patient's fears and wishes, to helping to give their last months meaning, to helping the caregivers deal with the process of grieving and loss.

PART TWO

DECISION-MAKING AND ETHICAL DECISIONS

Advanced Care Planning

Early on in life, most of us are taught that in many cases, in order to succeed, it is best to plan in advance for things. Whether the goal is to perform well on a test, to give an engaging presentation, or to organize a trip across a country, we have learned to anticipate obstacles and be prepared for challenges that come our way. Although we know this fact, there are certain situations where we'd rather not plan. Unfortunately, planning for care at the end of life can be a difficult, emotional task unlike any we have dealt with so far. Never mind planning—many family members and patients may even avoid or dread just *thinking* about planning for this difficult stage of life.

However, in order to ensure that end-stage dementia patients have the chance to receive the best care possible, family members shouldn't wait until their family member is facing imminent death. Instead, discussions with patients and families about end-of-life decisions and palliative approaches should take place early in the course of illness, ideally as early as the point of diagnosis.

An Ethical Approach

Before diving into specific issues concerning planning and communication, it may be helpful to review four key ethical principles that help frame the various ethical challenges and dilemmas that hospital ethicists, health care, and social service providers, as well as family members, will inevitably encounter along their journey of caregiving:

Respect for autonomy

This principle entails accepting the patient's right to **participate in the decision-making process that affects their medical treatment**. Within the process by which medical decisions are made, the patient's view, opinions, and wishes must be respected, and their choices cannot be ignored by those responsible for providing care. It is the consideration of the patient's perspective on their own care that provides them with the dignity they deserve when medical decisions are made and treatments considered. It is the duty of those responsible for making decisions on behalf of a loved one (as the *substitute decision-maker,* or SDM) to do it in good conscience, as they believe their loved one would want them to act (see Substitute Decision-making, pp. 30-31).

Non-maleficence

In general all steps should be taken to **avoid—or when this is not possible, to minimize—harm to a patient receiving medical care**. When a person is in the end stages of life, this principle's focus is to, whenever possible, avoid exaggerating any harm that is not necessary for care and, of course, to avoid intentionally inflicting harm. This might translate into decisions to avoid undertaking potentially painful or stressful medical tests that may offer minimal if any substantial benefit for the patient, such as blood tests, spinal taps, and X-rays or CT and MRI scans.

Beneficence

This has been the core of medical ethics for centuries: **the desire and commitment to help the patient and alleviate pain and suffering whenever possible**. Therefore, during the end-of-life situations, treatments should have some potential to help the patient in some domain of care. Health care and social service providers should have this as a *primary focus* of their collective efforts.

Justice

Health care professionals must treat patients equitably and fairly. It is not acceptable to decide who receives a scarce resource on the basis of characteristics such as gender, religious beliefs, age, social or economic status, or ethnicity. This principle guides the everyday reality of health care systems:

there will never be enough resources to treat everyone in an optimal manner. At the very least, we must ensure that unmerited and unnecessary treatments are limited as much as possible, so that patients who may significantly benefit can receive the necessary resources.

Communication

Talking with patients and families about end-of-life care should begin relatively early. Opening up the lines of communication right from the start means that there is a foundation where individuals can continue discussions as the illness advances and worsens. In other words, there shouldn't just be one long, detailed talk about end-of-life decisions at the beginning of the process, but rather a routine of end-of-life conversations structured as part of the many interventions. Both empirical evidence and clinical experience show that these continued discussions improve outcomes and adherence to the patients' wishes.

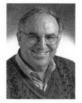

Dr. Gordon Discusses

I can highlight the consequences of not having these sorts of discussions by providing an example of two siblings who, as their mother's situation deteriorated, were at opposite ends of the interventions scale. The mother, in the end stage of dementia, was completely non-communicative, bed-bound, unable to eat, and unable to provide any self-care. The siblings agreed to not provide artificial nutrition and hydration in keeping with what they thought would be their mother's wishes. But, when she developed an infection, one sibling wanted her transferred to a general hospital and the other wanted her to stay and receive comfort care. Their approaches to the decisions would make one think that they were from different families.

As a result, their mother and the health care staff were caught in the middle of a difficult family conflict. This type of situation is much more common than you think; in fact, it might almost be considered the unfortunate norm.

Communication, long-term consideration, and planning by families are key to making sure that the end-of-life care issues are discussed and explored in order to maintain family peace and provide a dignified end for those we hold so dear.

First discussions can begin with the use of open-ended questioning in order to understand the patients' views on important issues such as illness, suffering, medical treatments, and death. Healthcare professionals may ask patients to talk a bit about themselves, and to talk about their past experiences with illness, doctors, and medical treatments. It is critical for the professionals to convey clearly that they will respect the patients' wishes and not abandon the patient ever, even when disease-focused treatments are no longer helpful or effective. This also is a good time to help the patient understand the concept of palliative care.

Ongoing conversations with the patient and family are also likely to include the topics explored further below.

Informed Consent

In the best case scenario, patients can still communicate their personal opinions about decisions that may come up in the course of their illness. Informed consent means that the patient has the necessary and sufficient information to comprehend what is involved in the decision and **can understand the potential and real consequences**. They must also be able to make that decision freely, which means there has not been undue influence from others. But informed consent still allows input and advice from loved ones.

In Canada there is an obligation to obtain informed consent for many types of health care interactions. Opinions have differed, though, regarding exactly what information should be shared with the patient. For example, in Ontario the Health Care Consent Act (1996) states that the information must include the following:

- The nature of the treatment;
- The expected benefits;
- The material risks and side effects associated with it;
- Alternative courses of action; and
- The likely consequences of not having treatment.

Caregivers and professionals should take measures to ensure that the information has been clearly communicated to the patient. They can clarify particular points and ask questions in order to assess understanding on behalf of the patient. It is also very useful to ask questions that clarify what values and beliefs that underlie their decisions, as this provides the opportunity to discuss other options for care and informs future decision-making.

Information Disclosure

Both the patient and family should be informed of relevant facts as the disease progresses. As complications occur and/or curative-focused treatments fail, it is important for the family to continue to be informed in a way that promotes a kind of partnership in decision-making. So, if there is bad news to deliver, health care workers should communicate this up-front and open the discussion on the goals of treatment. This can only take place if the parties involved are emotionally ready to engage in frank and realistic communication.

A simple approach is to tell the patient or family that unfortunately there is some bad news and then to ask if they would like to talk about this now. It is usually advisable to undertake such a discussion only after there have been a number of clinical interactions and it is believed that a strong therapeutic alliance has been established between patient and health care provider and/or family and health care provider. It is a judgment call on behalf of the health care provider, and probably family members, to determine that the necessary element of trust exists for such an important topic to be discussed. There should be a good comfort level where difficult questions naturally arise.

The family or the patient may inquire how long the patient has to live, for example. In this case, it may be helpful to respond first by conveying empathy for the process underlying the patient or family's statement. It is then important to convey the typical prognosis with the best knowledge available, the possible ranges of prognosis, and any clinically pertinent factors that may alter the prognosis. If the answer to a question is particularly bleak, health care professionals may also feel the need to "soften the blow" by acknowledging that there is always going to be certain degree of uncertainty in any illness trajectory. That said, it is the most helpful in the long term to put primary emphasis on being honest about whatever facts *are* known.

Capacity

A large part of respecting a patient's autonomy—and more broadly speaking, of practicing "patient-centred care"—is honouring the individual's right to participate in the decision-making process, even if others may not agree with these decisions. Determining when it is necessary to transfer this right from the patient to a designated representative known as a Substitute Decision Maker (SDM) becomes an ethical as well as legal task. In order to demonstrate their capacity to make informed decisions, patients should be able to comprehend the facts of their condition, appreciate the meaning of these facts, and express a choice based on a reasoned consideration of the situation in a manner congruent with his or her personal and cultural preferences and values.

It isn't always easy to assess capacity. Subtle cognitive difficulties may produce a state of "partial capacity," for example. A patient may experience a "lucid moment" where he or she is able to communicate preferences, and many agree that this may be used as a valid expression of capable preference or decision.

Capacity can also change as the patient's mental and cognitive state improves or worsens over time. For this reason, many have argued for a "sliding scale" approach to capacity determinations. This approach instructs that with medical decisions that are of low danger and in the patients' best interests, it is best to take a less stringent capacity standard. With very serious and potentially dangerous decisions, a stricter capacity standard should still be applied.

In ordinary practice, capacity is focused on medical decisions or decisions, for example, related to key elements of care, such as when it appears necessary to provide institutional care rather than to attempt to maintain care at home. When it comes to personal preferences related to food, clothes, or hygiene, which are not strictly speaking medical decisions, there is a general tendency to allow the greatest latitude possible. It is preferable to have the person make their own decisions, as long as these decisions do not generate substantial risk for harm. There are instances in which family members assume that if a personal decision—for example, related to food—is not in conformance with the highest standards of health promotion, they should find ways to prevent their loved one of partaking. One has to try to look at the broad picture in terms of what life has to offer and find ways to be less rigid and to promote as much personal well-being, satisfaction, and comfort as possible.

Substitute Decision-making

Families or caregivers should ask their loved ones if they have an up-to-date "living will," or an *advance directive*, that reasonably reflects their current wishes. The issue of *substitute decision-makers* (SDMs), or "proxy decision-makers," should also be **ideally discussed when the patient is cognizant enough to designate who they would like to take on this role.**

If an SDM is not identified, there is usually a legal definition, depending on the jurisdiction, of who is expected to take on the role. In Ontario, for example, in section 20 of the Health Care Consent Act, the role is designated to a spouse or partner, and if there is none, then a child or parent, then a brother, sister, or other relative. There are also usually criteria such as minimum age of sixteen and willingness to assume the responsibility. A SDM can also be specifically appointed by the courts.

This role of SDM is to be assumed when a loved one is no longer able to effectively communicate his or her wishes or no longer has the capacity for informed consent as described above. **The main job of the SDM by law is to respect any known previous wishes of their loved one.** These wishes may be identified through an advanced directive, through earlier conversations, or understood by cultural, religious, or personally expressed preferences. The actual decisions that are made by the SDM require the same elements of informed consent as the patient would have required.

If there is already an advanced directive, it should be respected, although in many situations, there is some interpretation of its terms that is required by the SDM. That is why it is usually recommended that individuals who have formulated an advance directive discuss its content and principles with their SDMs. Families will often find that it is easier to respect the "negative" versus "positive" wishes expressed in these directives; for example, "I don't want a feeding tube in the case of a severe stroke" versus "I want euthanasia in the case of a severe stroke." If the patient does not have an advance directive or cannot communicate his or her particular desires, the decision-makers must then decide in the best interest of their family member what should happen as the need for decisions arises. In order for the SDM to act appropriately and according to the intention of the concept and the law, they need to understand and accept that **they are not being asked to consider their own personal values, but rather what seems to be the preference of the patient**, or in general terms, what most people would probably want if a specific preference cannot be determined. They need to take into consideration all of the factors about the patient's condition and treatment alternatives, along with the known or presumed values, attitudes, and beliefs of the patient.

SDMs should ideally be supported by other caregivers and/or health care professionals while they carry out this substantial and often difficult responsibility. This shared decision-making process is an essential part of good care in patients with end-stage dementia. The family should be informed that they share the path of gradual deterioration together and that it is important to keep in contact. Health care professionals should be continually informing the family members about the prognoses and general course of the illness and the anticipated outcomes. This is helpful because it prepares the family for stressful situations and can help to ease decision-making.

Discussing Patient History

The patient should also be continually reassessed in terms of his or her symptoms (See Appendix A). Accordingly, they should be informed about any interventions, whether therapeutic or palliative in nature. Health care professionals should try to get specific information about physical and emotional symptoms while simultaneously seeing these in the broader context of the particular patient's illness history and trajectory.

Decision-Making

The importance of discussing the inevitable end-of-life decision-making early in the illness trajectory has been reiterated many times now. Often, big decisions, such as whether to pursue or continue curative-focused interventions (often consisting of mechanical ventilation and cardiopulmonary resuscitation, treatment of infections, and other intercurrent illnesses) are left to be discussed at the time of crisis rather than ahead of time. Of course, it is never easy to bring up these kinds of decisions in a more clinically stable period, but it is during this time when patients and their families can weigh the options. In times of emergency or crisis, most family members will intuitively want life-extending care. But if decision-making is discussed in advance, both patients and families are more likely to be in the frame of mind to absorb information regarding prognosis and then to make well-informed decisions accordingly. The palliative-care approach is usually the more likely choice if the clinical course of dementia is discussed along with the low likelihood of significant recovery after cardiopulmonary resuscitation and the substantial potential for further suffering.

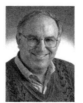

Dr. Gordon Discusses

The daughter was in turmoil. Her mother was suffering from late-stage dementia, and she and her two brothers could not agree on whether to put in a feeding tube. It was becoming impossible to provide adequate nutrition, as there had already been two episodes of aspiration pneumonia. "We are in complete disagreement, and I do not know what to do. I cannot accept that we can let her die like that." I asked her what she thought her mother would want under the circumstances.

"We never talked about such things. My brothers and I tried to bring up the topic, and she told us it was not something she wanted to discuss. She was a very proud woman and always had a positive view of the world. Talk of illness and dying were just too morbid for her."

I asked, "In the absence of actual discussions, what do you think she would want, knowing what kind of person she was?"

The daughter replied, "She was a tenacious person and always a fighter." I outlined some of the considerations she should bring into her and her siblings' decision-making process. These included whether or not her mother was particularly religious, how she dealt with personal pain and discomfort, how she reacted when other family or friends had illnesses from which they died, and what kind of comments she would make about the apparent suffering of others as examples that might reflect her values. Such observations might help the children understand and agree to what they thought would matter to their mother. I left it to the daughter to discuss these ideas with her siblings.

This discussion occurred a few days after a series of meetings I had attended in which challenges in long-term care planning by elders with their children was one of the topics of the program. Over and over again, the various eldercare specialists and planners that were gathered came back to the concept of "having the conversation." We all agreed that there was often an enormous reluctance for loved ones to broach the subject of future planning, ranging from living arrangements and financial planning preferences to expressing wishes for end-of-life or serious life-imperiling situations. The question that kept coming up was why there was such a reluctance to explore one's wishes and values when late-stage illnesses occur.

Many reasons were given by those sitting around the table, including superstition, discomfort in facing negative aspects of life, religious beliefs, one's personality, and difficulties in relationships. Some years ago, there was large-scale impetus for people to develop advance directives as a way of assuring their wishes would be honored. For some people, the process proved useful, whereas for others it became too complicated or threatening. From the studies of that process, many eldercare specialists concluded that the written document was not the most important part of the process; rather, it was **the conversation that explored wishes and personal values.** These conversations formed the basis of decisions that reflected what the person was likely to say if they could assist in the process.

The daughter I had spoken to called back a few weeks later and told me that she and her siblings decided against the feeding tube and allowed their mother to receive supportive and palliative care with comfort measures only for her last *weeks of life. She said, "I wish we had had the conversation, but I believe this is what our mother would have wanted." I counsel all those I can in clinical settings and in lectures to try to have that important conversation with loved ones so that decisions can be made during the last period of your life that reflect your wishes and values.*

Confidentiality, Privacy, and Respectfulness

Throughout the process of caring for patients with dementia, health care and social services will be privy to a lot of personal information. Some of this information may cover topics that the patient would not be willing to share with anybody else. This information is obviously to be kept confidential, as demanded by essentially all health care and social service workers' codes of ethics and privacy legislation in most jurisdictions. Personal information should only be shared with those individuals directly involved in the patient's care and who have a need to know. This strict code of confidentially is crucial in terms of respecting the patient's autonomy and sense of control. It also plays a large role in promoting mutual trust and clear communication in relationships between caregivers and patients.

Some methods to assure that confidentiality is protected include:

- Finding private, or relatively private, areas to have discussions with the patient;
- Not discussing patient information in public areas (e.g., cafeteria);
- Keeping health records in a secure, locked place; and
- Going to the patient to consult when there is a question about the appropriateness of sharing information for as long as they have the capacity to comment.

Expanding on the last point, it can be very hard to keep information from the patient's family, but if the patient *is* still able to communicate, many health care professionals and perhaps some lawyers argue that unless he or she has given permission either formally or informally, it isn't acceptable to discuss the patient's illness with family members. It is typically the case that family members *are* the main avenue of communication in terms of the patient's illness, but this still shouldn't be automatically assumed.

These issues should be discussed between health care professionals and patients early on in the patient's illness trajectory to establish the level of privacy and information sharing that he or she is comfortable with. In many situations, by the nature of the way clinical interactions have taken place, *implied* consent in such situations is usually sufficient to fulfill the test of *consent*. For example, family members frequently accompany their loved one to clinical visits, clearly in an agreed to fashion, where information is shared openly. When I first meet a patient that is accompanied by a family member and often a personal care worker, I usually ask if there is any problem with the family coming in to the interview with the patient. While I do not recall a situation where the patient has not consented, it is however a good baseline to establish, depending on the jurisdiction.

There are times where there is an unacceptable risk of harm to the patient or someone else where it is acceptable, legal, and in certain cases obligatory to breach confidentiality. These situations include:

- When the patient has a mental condition or illness that may lead to personal harm or harm to others. In this case, information should be revealed if necessary for proper care, public protection, and general safety, and only to those who are required to know to lessen the risk.
- When there is a reasonable suspicion of elder abuse. Cases like these should always be reported, but in many jurisdictions, individuals are required by law to report to the appropriate authorities.
- When the patient has a particular communicable/infectious disease that must be reported by law to the authorities. For example, Methicillin-resistant Staphylococcus aureus (MRSA), Clostridium Difficile, and influenza infections (all particularly common in long-term care settings) require certain care precautions that make confidentiality virtually impossible.

Nutrition and Hydration

One of the biggest ethical dilemmas in end-of-life care is related to nutrition and hydration. There are some patients who make the decision themselves to stop eating and drinking. In a palliative situation, this may be a result of the illness that reduces appetite and makes the process of eating very difficult or unpleasant, or the patient may have reached a point where they want to end their own suffering. In these cases, the patient still has the capacity to make an informed decision.

However, when a patient is simply unable to feed him or herself, it becomes the job of family members, close friends, or health care and social service providers to undertake the feeding process. There may come a time when the patient begins to resist being fed. At this point, family members or substitute decision-makers and health care professionals need to have a frank discussion about how they are going to provide nourishment to the patient, if at all.

Providing nutrition through a feeding tube requires a procedure to insert the feeding tube. Usually this goes without problems, but sometimes there can be complications from the tube, including leakage around the site of insertion or infection. Moreover, once a tube is in place, even if the SDM decides that they made an error in judgment in its insertion, its cessation often feels much more dramatic than not inserting it in the first place. Emotionally it may feel like actually "killing" the person when the tube feed is discontinued. This makes the decision about feeding and hydration a complicated issue where the opinions, wishes, experiences, and values of the patient, family members, and health care professionals should be carefully considered.

It might be helpful to families and health care providers to consider that the use of a feeding tube is generally and commonly used in the acute care system, intended as a short-term solution. This is usually for a patient who is expected to recover to a state where they can again swallow food, or as an assistive device to address new complications of a disease where the patient is otherwise able to maintain a reasonable quality of life. This is especially important to consider with patients with end-stage dementia, as such patients are not expected to recover to a point where they can again swallow food and fluids, and not providing nutrition does not negatively impact on their quality of life, especially if they are refusing adequate nutrition by mouth.

The same can be said about artificial hydration (usually intravenous or subcutaneous fluids). This issue is a bit tricky because intuitively most family members consider artificial hydration a kind of comfort provision for their loved one, a measure used to prevent them from dying an uncomfortable death from dehydration. Nowadays, most experts agree that in the majority of cases, the negative impact and harms of artificial hydration may exceed the benefits for the person who is in late-stage dementia.

Fortunately many good health care institutions have a lot of information that thoroughly discusses the pros and cons of artificial nutrition and hydration. These resources should be shared and discussed with patients and family members, ideally before this issue arises. **Of special note is that artificial nutrition and hydration does not decrease the likelihood of aspiration and resultant pneumonia, rarely improves nutritional status, only sometimes prolongs life for any substantial period of time, and has no beneficial impact on quality of life or on the quality of the dying process.**

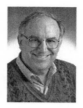

Dr. Gordon Discusses

It started with a phone call. "I need your advice about whether or not we should put a feeding tube into my father." It was the mother of one of our children's friends. "He had a very bad stroke and has recovered, and is in an acute care hospital awaiting placement. He cannot eat, and we have had two conflicting opinions about putting in the tube. My brother and I do not know what to do."

It is a common scenario played out in hospitals all over world. Depending on the jurisdiction and the ethno-cultural-religious views of those involved, the issue can be tilted one way or the other. For those who subscribe to religions that espouse the "sanctity of life," it is almost deemed obligatory to put in a feeding tube (medically called a gastrostomy tube or G-tube, requiring a procedure called a Percutaneous Endoscopic Gastrostomy, or PEG procedure). For those who espouse the "quality-of-life" perspective, the procedure might be rejected if, in the opinion of the potential recipient or their surrogate, it does not add any substantial comfort.

Many families express concerns about the experience of hunger or sense of starvation if a feeding tube is not provided. Most of the evidence available supports the observation that as long as proper mouth care is provided to avoid dryness of the mucous membranes and lips, the true sensation of hunger does not occur and the process does not lead to the experience of starvation or suffering. The body is very adept at protecting itself from such physical experiences, and in the absence of food for a prolonged period, produces chemicals known as ketones that blunt the hunger sensation.

There are the many individuals who have no fixed personal, religious, or culturally dominant view who are open to considering all medical procedures as long as they know and understand the implications of the proposed treatment.

There are some health care professionals, such as Dr. Susan Mitchell of Harvard University, who have interpreted the medical literature on the subject as indicating that it does little in terms of long-term benefit. There are those, in contrast, who contend that although it does not achieve its goals in all circumstances, it does maintain life in many who would otherwise succumb to inanition (progressive weight loss and what in essence is a state of starvation).

I am frequently consulted by families and health care staff when a decision has to be made to insert a feeding tube or attempt feeding with a modified and "safer" diet. An approach that I use takes into account clinical, personal, cultural, religious, and family views on the matter. The important clinical question is that in some conditions, there will be progressive and unrelenting deterioration such that a feeding tube is merely a "stop-gap" in the process and may not really change the actual course of the disease. In other conditions, the disease may stabilize and artificial feeding may prolong life for an undefined and sometimes extensive period. This latter outcome is very unusual in late-stage dementia, as the condition is most often unrelenting in its progressive deterioration.

Many experts in the field have studied the impact of artificial nutrition and hydration. They have come to the conclusion that because of the important symbolism of "food and drink," it can be very helpful if families, with the help of the nursing staff and dieticians, are offered the option of **conscientious hand-feeding**, *as noted by Gillick and Mitchell of Harvard University. This means that with proper instruction by the professional staff, whatever oral intake that can be managed is offered to the person experiencing the last stages of dementia. When such a program is undertaken, it should be accepted that whatever is taken in will be sufficient to fulfill the symbolic aspect of feeding. Even if the nutritional requirements are not met, that is not as important as the symbolism associated with the process of feeding by caring staff and loved ones. With such undertakings, tube feeding, which rarely has a true extended beneficial impact on the person and has many negative aspects to it, can be avoided without family members feeling guilty about what might be perceived as abandonment of a basic need of a loved one.*

Sometimes the question of stopping intravenous (IV) hydration comes up when the patient is close to the end of life. The family feels they would be depriving their loved one of fluids, leading them to a premature death. It is very important to explain that in the process of dying, the body can no longer use the fluids and providing them may cause fluid retention (edema), which increases suffering and aggravates breathing difficulties. Also, it is important to dispel the myth that by discontinuing IV fluids, the person will feel thirsty. Those providing care must instead emphasize good mouth care, in which the membranes of the lips and mouth are kept moistened by swabbing with specialized moisturizers. This is a very simple thing to do and is again a comforting task for loved ones who are at the bedside.

The next issue is what the family believes the person would have wanted if they were able to give their views on the matter. Often, family members who are substitute decision makers forget or do not understand that their role in decision-making is to reflect what they, in good conscience, believe their loved one would have wanted if they could make the decision themselves. The personal view of the decision-maker should not be what governs the decision.

When there are religious views held by the patient, they must be interpreted by the surrogate, sometimes with the assistance of religious advisors to determine "what is right" in that religion's view. At the end, a decision has to be made, but it is important to remember that in most North American jurisdictions, decisions such as these can be legally reversed and artificial feeding discontinued if there is reason to believe that it is the best and most appropriate choice after it has been tried for a period of time. It may not feel good to make such a decision, but sometimes it is the best decision to make under the circumstance, especially when the hoped-for improvement does not occur and it appears that suffering has not been allayed nor function or comfort improved. By continuing to offer even small amounts of food and drink by mouth, even in the very late stages of dementia, feelings of guilt by family members can be assuaged.

Pain and Other Symptoms

The main goal of palliative care is the relief of symptoms, such as pain and shortness of breath, to promote optimal comfort. Though this may read as a simple objective, it can present a large moral dimension for many people involved in the care of a patient. For example, health care and social service providers may not agree about the amount of analgesic medication that should be given. Some caregivers may feel that they are not able to provide optimal palliative care without seeming to be ending a patient's life prematurely.

It must be recognized that **it is ethically acceptable, and even obligatory, to provide pain and other symptom relief at the patient's or substitute decision-maker's request**. There was a time when there were concerns expressed that the provision of such treatments, especially pain medications, could potentially shorten the patient's life. If this were the case, it would be understandable from an emotional and/or spiritual or religious perspective that it could be very difficult for some individuals to accept palliative care. Most of the evidence now appears to indicate that proper attention to and treatment of symptoms such as pain does not alter the trajectory of dying. It is unusual for such medications to shorten life when given according to usually accepted protocols and standards, which often entail gradual adjustments of the dosage. Some patients prefer to tolerate a certain level of pain or discomfort in order to avoid the sedating effects of some medications.

When substitute decision-makers (SDM) are making decisions about pain relief, there may be conflicts between that individual and the health care team about appropriate scheduling or amounts of medication. A helpful process to follow in this situation should ideally include:

- Exploring the reasoning for the SDM's decisions and explaining the health care and social service providers' concerns.
- Following up on the SDM's reasoning or concerns. Is the substitute having difficulty with the impending death of their loved one? What would their loved one want?
- Determining whether the health care and social service provider believe that the SDM is not acting on the request of the patient nor in the patient's best interests. If so, outside help (e.g., legal intervention or the hospital ethicist) may be beneficial.
- Exploring whether the SDM realizes the need for treating the pain and that denying treatment will cause suffering.

Sometimes it is the health care providers who have a problem realizing that there is a need to treat pain in a patient who is cognitively impaired, or they may not recognize that the cause of behavioural symptoms in the patient might be due to unrecognized and therefore untreated pain.

Withholding or Stopping Life-Sustaining Treatments

A challenging aspect of caring for patients with end-of-life dementia is the decision to withhold or withdraw life-sustaining, or what appear to be life-sustaining, treatments. Many professionals these days are starting to argue that these treatments are medically futile (usually meant in ethics writings as *a medical conclusion or determination that a therapy is of no value to a patient and should not be prescribed).* This is a contentious issue because it could easily be argued that whether something has value or not is dependent on the eye of the beholder. For example, to some family members, a short time of survival may have great value, while to the health care team, it may seem unwarranted and of little benefit.

When health care and social service providers are reluctant to agree to treatments that patients or families want, it may be because they have a profound sense that further treatment would be fundamentally wrong. It is only by open communication between patients, family members, and health care and social service providers that treatment decisions can be reached. If one relies on the view that a treatment is futile or has acquiesced to requests for additional interventions, the result may be further avoidance of the honest discussion of the patient's prognosis and alternatives for treatment.

An excellent example is the changing attitudes toward cardiopulmonary resuscitation (CPR). At some stages of life, and in certain situations of illness, CPR is considered standard if someone were to have a cardiac or pulmonary arrest. However, more recently, there is substantial evidence to suggest that CPR may have little to offer patients who have various medical problems and are also experiencing the later stages of dementia.

Accordingly some individuals may choose a "do not resuscitate" option or goal (a DNR order) as part of their decision-making plan. This is the kind of important, literally life-changing request that should be discussed in advance with family and health care professionals. There are many resources (see Resources section) that can be used to help educate all parties involved and stimulate discussion about decision-making earlier in the illness trajectory. Unlike the media's erroneous representation of CPR, where most individuals appear to respond, benefit, and survive, in the elderly frail population—especially in those who have lived with dementia for many years and are in the last stages of life—the procedure falls into the category of futile. It results in what is in essence a last, most undignified, and intrusive undertaking. It is likely to be painful (though we rarely can verify this, as the vast majority of people undergoing CPR in such circumstances die). Even if successful, CPR could not leave the person with any semblance of quality of life, and it merely postpones death for an extremely short period.

Dealing with Conflict

It isn't surprising that conflict often arises around providing versus not providing life-sustaining care in late- or terminal-stage dementia. Ideally, care decisions are guided by the patient's values, beliefs, and culture, with consideration of medical best practices and evidence-based information. But it is understandable that conflict arises.

Sometimes conflict is the result of differences in cultural, ethnic, or religious orientation and values. As we experience an increase in multiculturalism and people with a wide range of values, it is natural and expected that sometimes conflicts occur because of different value systems. When these values impact on health care decisions, there is sometimes a breakdown in understanding, empathy, and communication that can lead to conflict and animosity. Some of the issues related to differences in value systems will be addressed in Part Three of this book.

While it is unrealistic to expect everyone to agree in order to work together, there *should* be an expectation of mutual respect in a health care setting. Even though health care professionals may feel like they hold the knowledge and power to perhaps persuade the family of the "correct" steps to take in order to properly care for the patient, they must, at the very least, take the time to listen and try to understand the wishes of all parties involved. So, once again, always trying to promote clear communication between the patient, family, and health care professionals is a key preventative step to beginning or worsening conflict.

There may also be conflicts within health care teams. Although it seems worrisome and unprofessional to present these differences to the patient's family, the silver lining in this situation is that the team's conflict opens up communication by allowing families to feel more comfortable in expressing their own conflicts and differences in opinion. While it can be challenging, my experience of such an approach, as long as communication occurs in a respectful manner, has fostered improved trust by the family, an increased sense of value and respect amongst team members, and improved care for the patient.

If a conflict becomes very complicated and seems to be getting out of hand, it may be useful to use an ethical framework or consult with an ethicist or mediator. For those institutions that can support such a role even part-time, a medical ethicist can be an invaluable reference point and a neutral party to aid decision-making in a crisis, as well as providing proactive education on a ongoing basis. This approach generally fosters a basic level of understanding and a common language when there are differences of opinion.

Summary

- Ethical issues in late-stage dementia are often about trying to achieve a balance between the element of autonomy, the patient's expressed preferences, and the patient's best interests (or at least what we would consider their best interest), along with other factors that may appear to be in conflict with those principles.
- While interventions that ease pain and breathing difficulties are largely beneficial, medical interventions such as tube-feeding, hydration, and CPR should be carefully considered, as they are rarely appropriately indicated.
- The more families and health care professionals openly communicate and engage in a dialogue about these issues, particularly in the early stages of the illness, the closer they may get to assuring that the decisions made are consistently acceptable to everybody involved.
- When an impasse is reached in terms of decision-making, it is most often helpful to get external guidance and assistance from someone who is not immediately connected to the situation, such as an ethicist or social worker, who can help explore the areas of conflict and work towards an acceptable resolution.

PART THREE

Comfort Care in Context

End of Life through Different Cultural Lenses

Canada is often referred to as a "cultural mosaic," a country where diversity is practiced and celebrated. It is safe to say that Canadians generally are able to maintain their original culture and ethno-cultural ties while at the same time integrating into the larger, evolving environmental culture. The situation of people from different cultures who maintain this duality is very important to consider in the context of end-of-life care. Patients and their families are coming from particular life narratives and perspectives; accordingly, the delivery of care should at least recognize this, if not be modified to accommodate it. Such cultural complexity exists in other countries as well, especially the United States, although there the approach to the absorption of immigrants has been traditionally one of the "melting pot" rather than the "cultural mosaic" model.

The way someone experiences treatment and healing is very much influenced by their culture. Significant life passages like death and the process of dying are also handled differently depending on an individual's culture and religion. Each culture has special understandings and rituals associated with the process of dying, and it would be ideal for health care institutions to foster an environment where expression of culture is both respected and encouraged.

At the same time, one of the cornerstones of palliative care and practice is considering every patient as a unique individual to be respected. So although people are in part a product of their cultural group, they shouldn't simply be expected to behave in certain ways and believe certain things because of their cultural heritage. It is all about being sensitive to both the patient's cultural group and the individual's idiosyncrasies, and finding the equilibrium between the two.

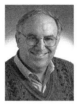

Dr. Gordon Discusses

It was the second time in less than a month that a request came to assist families struggling with decisions about loved ones in serious end-of-life situations. The circumstances were similar. Both families were struggling with whether or not to "let go" and if so how. One parent was in an intensive care unit and one in a regular unit in an acute hospital. The outlook for both appeared dismal from the perspective of the medical staff that, according to the families, had done everything reasonably possible to save the life of their loved one. But things had not gone well, and now the end was growing near.

"We want to do the 'right thing,' not just as a family, but 'Jewishly.'" In both families, the degree of observance was modest but the reverence for Jewish values and traditions was high. They had received some input from rabbis but were struggling with whether the direction they received truly reflected the values they shared as a family and reflected the values of their loved one. Not an easy challenge for a devoted and loving family.

The question for me was what I might offer in my role as geriatrician and one who had done postgraduate studies in ethics. I understood the limitations of my background and training but was also aware of the many situations I had witnessed and my great interest in and respect for the teachings and values within Judaism. I knew that, not being a rabbi, my views were a secularized composite of the cases I had observed and the education I had been involved with over many years of practice. The challenge was mainly at the human level: the struggle with the notion of "letting go" of a beloved member of the family.

How a family deals with such heart-wrenching dilemmas can be addressed from many perspectives: the ethical, the legal, and the personal/familial. Ethically, most families want to do the "right" thing. Their understanding of the ethical approach to such decisions is usually a reflection of the principles and values on which they were raised. If there is a Jewish (strongly religious or not) component to such values, one hears often that families do not want any suffering for their loved one. Such concerns are fairly universal across all religions and ethnic groups. Families often struggle with concepts of duties to provide food and drink, often translated into the more clinical "nutrition and hydration," but the association with the loving act of feeding often cannot be disregarded. Promoting sanctity of life, a common theme in the three monotheistic religions, often competes with the secular concept of quality of life and avoidance of suffering.

Ontario law, similar to that in most North American jurisdictions, expects family or formally designated SDM decisions to reflect what they believe their loved one would have truly wanted or, when this is not possible to determine, what would be in their loved ones' "best interests." Many family members or SDMs do not truly know their loved one's wishes but may have some direct or indirect idea about their values. But true, explicitly expressed wishes are often not usually discussed; it is at the human level that the real challenge exists. Time is needed to discuss and explore feelings and values. At some point, it becomes necessary to make a difficult decision. I often counsel families that whatever decision they make, it is the "right one," whatever the outcome. Second guessing afterwards with "what ifs" is a terrible process that can lead to lifelong doubts and recriminations. Talk and feel and share as a family, and then make the best decision that you can. That is all any loving family can do.

Cultural Influence

Many key components of late-stage dementia care philosophy and practice can be influenced by a patient and family's culture and background. Some great questions to ask, or at least get indirect answers for, include:

- How important was religion in the life of your loved one?
- How consistent was your loved one in formal religious observance?
- What did your loved one express when important people, such as relatives, acted in a way contrary to traditional religious beliefs or values?
- Did your loved one consult with religious leaders or read books or magazines on religious issues?
- Did religious issues come up often during conversations when friends and family gathered?
- Did your loved one attend their house of worship on a regular basis?

Sometimes there appears to be a gap in the understanding of approaches to care and decision-making because of religious or ethno-cultural belief systems or practices. It is incumbent on those providing care to find ways of understanding the underlying principles particular religious or ethno-cultural groups so that appropriately sensitive decision support can be provided. Some key questions that may raise cultural, religious, or ethnic implications and practices include:

- **The patient and family as a unit of care:** How important is the family unit in this culture? What is the typical or accepted level of involvement in the patient's illness trajectory? What are the typical gender roles in this culture?
- **Certain physical aspects of care:** What is the role of physical touch? Is this person from a culture of strict physical privacy? What are dietary and nutritional requirements of this cultural group?
- **Symptom control:** How do this person and their family handle pain and pain control? What are their beliefs and values surrounding this issue? Are there certain complementary or alternative therapies that are traditionally used in this culture for the healing process?
- **Communication:** What are the roles of sharing emotions and talking in this culture? How about truth-telling about a patient's prognosis? Is there a language barrier? Are there ways that you could communicate using universal nonverbal cues?
- **Setting goals of care:** Would patients and families find the person-centered/collaborative approach to decision-making and care a bit frightening if they come from a culture where individual autonomy is not integral to the way their society functions?
- **Expressions of grief and mourning:** What is typical behaviour for those mourning and those visiting? What is appropriate to eat, drink, and wear in this culture?

Summary

- Palliative care, as laid out in this guide, is rooted in comfort, care, and compassion.
- It is only natural that being sensitive to the particular beliefs, values, and wishes of patients and their families would be understood as a key component of good practice in the delivery of care to individuals in late-stage dementia. Health care professionals must be sensitive to the cultural diversity of those that they care for.
- It is important to recognize gaps in understanding and take all necessary steps to bridge the ethno-cultural-religious gaps in communication, responsiveness, and practice.

Caring for the Caregiver

Emotional Distress

It is generally assumed that a loved one moving into a care home lowers the stress of family caregivers. While this may be true in terms of taking off some of the pressure for families in assisting with daily routines and responding to their family members' every single need, many individuals may experience new kinds of stressors. They may feel a new dimension of loss and grief, believing that they have taken their loved one out of a familiar home environment; they may worry about the level of care that is delivered by the staff of the care institution; and they can experience a relative loss of control or mastery compared to when they themselves were the primary caregivers.

There is also often a *caregiver burden,* defined by the Oxford Textbook of Palliative Medicine as "the emotional and physical demands and responsibilities of one's illness that are placed on family members, friends, or other individuals involved with the patient outside the health care system" (2003). Of importance is the fact that caregiver burden can exist even when the person being cared for is within the health care system. Loved ones continue to take on many tasks that can be exhausting, including visiting often, especially when long travel distances are involved; assisting their loved one with activities such as feeding, going for walks, or being taken around in a wheelchair; being involved in what is often emotionally stressful decision-making; and communicating with various health care providers and other members of the family. This burden can be impacted by a number of different factors, including culture, gender, coping style, social network, the number of family members who need care, and the caregiver's history or natural relationship with their loved ones. Learning to care for the caregiver is so important because this kind of distress and burden can lead to many serious problems, such as:

- Caregivers not paying enough attention to their own health, resulting frequently in mental illness (depression is more common in caregivers than in the general population);
- Increased strain on relationships within the family unit; and
- Financial strain related to medical bills, reduced income, interruption in employment, and health care facility living expenses.

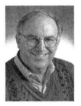

Dr. Gordon Discusses

"Sometimes you can't plan because the person you are planning for does not want any part of it." The husband of a colleague was told by a health care professional that there is really no planning he can undertake because his slightly cognitively impaired mother is adamant about not leaving her home. The son said, "There must be something I can do right now, even if my mother absolutely refuses anything I offer her. She understands up to a point but is so stubborn that I just can't move forward. I am very frustrated—I feel I should do something to plan for the future."

In a similar situation, two daughters visited my office with their father, who had many medical complaints—all of which were amenable to some beneficial intervention. However, as these were being discussed, including the issue of some depressive symptoms, one of the daughters said, "It is because of the situation at home. My mother is so stubborn and makes things very hard for my father. She refuses any help in the house and still expects him, at ninety-two, to take care of everything."

The daughters acknowledged that they were doing many of the ordinary tasks with their parents, including bill paying and household upkeep. Because their mother refused outside help other than them, they rotated with another sister and brother who would share in chores rotationally. "It works, but it is exhausting, and we see the frustration on my father's face every time we try and provide some sort of outside help and she rejects it. Her memory is poor, so sometimes the same issues come up repeatedly. She refuses to see doctors, so we cannot even find out if some medication might help. She not only fails to take her pills, but keeps telling my father he should stop taking his as well."

Such stories are not unusual and, for caring children, can be an awful dilemma, trying to figure out what to do while respecting their parent's wishes, even if they seem irrational. Even if legally one could remove the decision-making capacity from the parent by reason of mental incapacity, very few children are willing to "force" the parent into doing something they vehemently oppose. While many elderly individuals initially refuse a move to a long-term care facility, in practice many do get moved out of necessity, against what appears to be their wishes, and they adjust rather well.

However, sometimes the children must accept that they cannot force the situation but should keep trying whatever they can think of to cajole, induce, or convince their parent to try something different. At times, the children just have to wait things out until something happens that causes a crisis that requires intervention, and from there can move things forward. The important thing is to recognize that one cannot feel guilty because that is the way it worked out. As for the son that "wants to do something," I suggested he could explore long-term care facilities so that if and when the time comes, he knows what is available and what might be the best move, without having to explore this option under duress. The important thing to remember is that one can only do what can be done, and it is the caring that matters, even when the doing doesn't go exactly as one might want.

The Process of Caregiving

Staff and family members should try to work together right from the beginning of the caregiving process. Depending on the place in which end-of-life care is being provided, there initially may be some tension experienced by family members in handing over a lot of the responsibilities of a primary caregiving role to a set of strangers. This can be the case whether the care is being provided in the home, a hospice, a palliative care unit, a long-term care home, or any other venue. However, rather than having the dynamic play out as competitive, it is much more helpful to partner with the health care providers, remembering that the goal of providing care and comfort to their loved one will best be achieved this way.

If the individual requiring care is in a institutional setting, even one in which they have been for some period, the family can benefit from knowing how the facility operates within the context of end-of-life care, and more specifically what roles the various staff members have and who they can go to with concerns should they come up during this process. This small act can be empowering and may build or rebuild some feelings of mastery and control over the situation. Another way of forming a collaboration of care between health care professionals and family members, regardless of care setting, is to establish a routine for the family members. This should be the case whether the patient is living at home or in a long-term care or retirement home. Whenever possible, whatever the arrangement, family and friends should be involved somehow in the caregiving process. For example, if a daughter comes to visit her father in a long-term care home, she can assist with feeding and provide some interactive support by herself or along with others, depending on the situation. She might, for example, participate in a group music program along with her father.

I have always found that family members who participate in their loved one's daily routine almost always find it rewarding and come to think of the health care team as part of a new extended family. It is in these situations where the health care system can best provide care not only to the patient but to their caregiver. And it is those caregivers who come regularly that sometimes have their own illnesses detected early. Staff members recognize the early warning signs and feel comfortable approaching the caregiver because they have come to know them so well through their devoted caregiving efforts.

Loss and Grief

In many ways, bereavement can begin years before the actual death of a loved one. While dementia progresses slowly, it almost immediately interferes with full involvement and communication with those who care for them. This sense of grief then often increases as more and more losses and deficits occur. The grieving processes may start before the actual decision is made for palliative care or at any stage along the trajectory of the terminal stage of the illness. The most profound sense of loss may occur at points when major decisions are made, such as when artificial nutrition and hydration might be considered and then rejected, and the time period when the actual end of life can be anticipated. It can be particularly painful when the patient no longer recognizes family members and other close loved ones, which can happen at various points in the dementia trajectory.

Many family members find themselves in denial about the harsh realities of this illness. They may feel anger, shame, or self-pity, and also pity for their loved one as they recognize the degree of their cognitive and physical deterioration. It is important that everyone involved in a patient's care watch for and recognize the signs of grief and provide the appropriate support in a timely way.

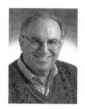

Dr. Gordon Discusses

I have heard it many times, from patients or family members: "I can't bear the thought of people seeing me (or him/her) like this." Sometimes the sentiment becomes a barrier to participating in programs or activities that might be very beneficial to the person and provide relief for family members.

I have seen individuals deprived of the potential benefit of attending day programs for seniors with cognitive impairment because the family was concerned that someone might recognize their loved one and realize that they have become afflicted with dementia. The family member might express a sense of "shame" at the thought that their beloved, previously highly respected member of the community, might be seen in a state of dependence, unable to express their wondrous lifetime of accomplishments.

Over the years, I have been involved in the care of numerous prominent individuals who have been afflicted with dementia or other conditions that have compromised their cognitive function and/or behaviour. Sometimes members of the staff involved in care know of the person's prominence, or may have some notion of their previous accomplishments. In contemporary long-term care homes, there is often an attempt to provide some place for memorabilia related to the resident's life and interests. It is often a useful way of engaging the person in discussions about their life, where distant memories are often preserved even in the face of the inability to retain or remember new information.

I recall one prominent physician I had known quite well during my academic career with whom I sat during the course of a centre-wide power failure. There was some recognition of who I was, and during the meanderings of our conversation, I was asked, "And how are you doing?"

I answered "Fine" and elaborated on activities that I believed he might be able to relate to, as they had involved him in the past. He listened carefully and actually made some comments that were relevant, even if somewhat tangential. The fact that he asked the same question of me ten minutes later, to which I responded in a like manner, did not matter. The important thing for me, and for him, is that we had a conversation that included important aspects of his life to which he could relate, even for some minutes.

Tragically, illnesses such as dementia of the Alzheimer's and other types do not choose those they afflict based on who that person is. Even with all the steps that we are told to undertake to decrease the risks of these diseases, about one-third of individuals over the age of eighty-five years will likely be affected. How our families cope with the implications of the illness and the years of gradual decline and dependency are the real challenges. One thing, however, I can encourage is that one should not allow pride and vanity to interfere with steps that might provide a beneficial interaction or activity on the part of one's loved one. I recall seeing a picture of the late President Ronald Reagan raking leaves, a task he could apparently do based on long-remembered rote tasks, and that gave him some satisfaction.

The key message for families is: move beyond your need for pride and accept the reality for what it is. Make every moment and any opportunity for meaningful interactions, however limited, available for your loved one and for those devoted to and caring for him/her.

Transcendence: Different Ways of Connecting

At this point, caregivers may find it helpful to take some alternative approaches in order to relate to their loved one. The patient may not be able to recognize others or communicate with words, but there are ways that caregivers can help to transcend these challenges. When patients with late-stage dementia become immobile and almost completely dependent, it can be easy to forget their psychological or spiritual needs because their physical needs are so apparent. Depending on the patient, a way to connect may be through the senses.

Touch: Caregivers may want to hold the patient's hand, brush his or her hair, or even give a gentle massage to the hands, legs, or feet. This tactile experience can be very meaningful for both patient and caregiver. If the caregiver is uncomfortable with the idea of providing massage, it may be worthwhile arranging for someone who is trained in massage therapy to provide a suitable level of massage to the ill person.

Smell: The patient may find pleasure in a favourite perfume, flower, or food. If it is a matter of a favourite food, and if the person is still able to take food by mouth, combining the aromatic smells with taste can be very satisfying and bring back pleasurable associations.

Hearing: Reading can be comforting and soothing even if the patient can't understand the words. Music is also very well known to bring comfort to individuals at all stages of cognitive decline. It is important that the music be chosen based on the known preferences of the person. Sometimes the use of personal music devices with earphones may enhance the musical experience, as it makes it very personal with no distractions; at other times, music within the context of a group may be more effective.

Sight: Nature images and videos may be relaxing for people in late-stage dementia. Here it is important to choose visual stimulation that is known to have been pleasing to the person in the past and can be readily accessed by them in a suitable context. Noisy television images may have a negative effect, but a previously loved movie in a quiet environment might be appreciated, even if it is not believed that the person may be able to appreciate all aspects of the film.

Coping with Grief

Although grief is an understandable and very normal part of the experience of dementia for both the person with dementia and his or her family, it can often be difficult for health care professionals to be open about these kinds of issues. Death as a topic of conversation is generally avoided until it is absolutely necessary to address. There are multiple barriers that prohibit the expression of grief amongst health care professionals, including when they are part of institutional staff. In particular, many caregiving professionals think that it is best to maintain a "proper" and professional distance. Even though the nature of their work makes confronting end-of-life issues inevitable, some health care professionals may demonstrate a lack of legitimacy for grieving, referred to as "disenfranchised grief" (Moss et al., 2003). In such cases, the health care professional may not legitimize or appreciate losses in what might appear to be a particularly sensitive manner. The loss is not openly acknowledged and so, in a way, family members can come to feel like their own grief and loss is not validated or supported.

Part of the reason that some health care professionals may take this seemingly cold approach is that they are probably being confronted with the death of their patients on a regular basis and so, in order to cope with the overload of loss in their lives, they have to maintain a certain level of detachment. This may not be the most effective way to cope with what appears to be excessive stress but, unless there is a system of support for such health care professionals, they may not be able to fully meet the needs of those they care for as well as their own personal and family needs, and their stress-laden work experience may spill over into their personal lives.

Though it seems like a logical coping mechanism from their perspective, it must be extremely difficult for family members who may be experiencing an immense amount of suffering (which feels very unique and painful to them) to be met with apparent unemotional coolness or distance from the health care professionals. Instead, professionals should aim to strike the right balance between maintaining a calm and perhaps a somewhat detached interior while still showing an appropriate amount of empathy and compassion on the exterior. They can convey this empathy through:

- Voice (tone, volume, speed, choice of words);
- Face (expression and eye contact should be appropriate for the situation); and
- Body language (some physical contact in certain circumstances may be suitable, such as a hug or gentle pat).

Summary

- There is a need for education and support for those who provide care for people with dementia.
- Stresses on the family continue even after a move to a health care, hospice, or palliative care setting, and may become particularly pronounced around the end of the patient's life.
- The caregiving role is vital to the delivery of quality care to patients with late-stage dementia.
- Though it does come with a set of burdens and challenges, caregiving can also enhance relationships, and many find the journey of caregiving a rewarding, meaningful, and even a spiritually enhancing experience.
- There are ways to find support and assistance in the caregiving role which can extend for a prolonged period. Caregivers should seek help so that they can cope with the challenges associated with the caregiving role.

A Sense of Autonomy

Taking the Perspective of the Patient

It is best to think of "person-centred care" as an approach or philosophy to providing care, rather than any one technique or therapeutic intervention. This approach is based on a core group of principles and values that can guide professional care providers (as well as family members and close friends) as to what should be done and how to go about doing it. This can be broken down into four main components (Brooker et al., 2004).

1. *Affirm the value of the person and their life, regardless of degree of impairment.*

For patients whose cognitive abilities have been severely diminished, this point is especially salient. Dementia undermines qualities that in Western society are often considered to be the things that make us distinctively human. These include coherent communication, memory, being socially-oriented, and having behavioural self-control (Jennings, 2004). Patients in late-stage dementia who can no longer remember their recent past may seem to have lost connection to their selves, and because of this lack of personal coherence, people around them may stop treating them like a person, whether they realize it or not.

Patients in late-stage dementia can begin to be perceived by those around them as being not fully alive or not fully human. This is often manifest by the common occurrence when people, including health care professionals, tend to talk *about* the person rather than to the person or including them in any group conversation, such as may occur at physician visits when the patient and family may be sitting in the office together.

Person-centred care requires a moral basis of care provision, which means acknowledging that the individual is a member of the human community who deserves attention and respect. Care should continue to be delivered in a personalized manner, even if the patient cannot fully communicate and participate in everyday activities.

2. *Treat everyone as an individual.*

This statement asserts that each individual with dementia is a unique human with a distinctive personality and personal history. When providing person-centred care, it is important to learn something about their past, to understand and delve into their personal narrative. Remember:

- This can be achieved by engaging in life history reviews with the patients if they can still communicate and/or with their close family members and friends.
- A patient's biography does not simply need to be written records, but can also include photographs, music, personal artifacts/objects, etc.
- The more health care providers apply the knowledge they have gained through narrative work with the patient and/or their families, the more individualized or person-centred care can be ensured.

3. *Adopt the perspective of the person with dementia.*

The person-centred approach starts with the underlying philosophy of seeing through the eyes of the person with dementia. This essentially means that family members and caregivers must come to recognize that each person's experience has its own psychological validity and that people with dementia act from, and because of, this particular perspective.

Looking at and understanding someone's subjective experience becomes a much more difficult task to accomplish when working with people with end-stage dementia. A lack of verbal expression by the person can make him or her harder to understand, and it can also be difficult to try and relate to a person when they don't seem to be lucid or have awareness. Steven R. Sabat, in his wonderful book *The Experience of Alzheimer's Disease: Life Through a Tangled Veil* (2001), provides wonderful insights into the challenges of communicating by and with persons living with dementia, and it provides guidance for caregivers to enhance the ability to communicate with those they love, despite severe communication difficulties.

4. *Provide a supportive social environment.*

This means that people with dementia should not only be viewed in terms of their behavioural and cognitive functioning, but as social, spiritual, emotional, and physical beings. It is also important to note that although the person-centred care approach is constantly emphasizing the concept of the individual, there are other congruent approaches that put the idea of relationships and interdependence at the forefront of their models of care. In relation-centred care, proposed by Nolan et al. (2004), the emphasis is on trying to further supportive social conditions. The patient's environment is examined and adjusted to improve the caregiving process, with the key people in his or her life being involved.

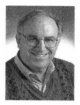

Dr. Gordon Discusses

Imagine arriving at the doctor's office because your throat hurts. The doctor touches your glands and asks if it hurts. You nod, and the doctor proceeds to take a swab knowingly and already anticipates that you may have a case of strep throat. Similarly, if you have been suffering with migraines and decide to seek professional help, a physician may ask you where exactly you feel this head pain, what the "quality" of pain feels like, and to what degree you are feeling it—is it a throbbing dull pain or a sharp, spurt-like, intense pain? In these cases, alleviating pain is quickly and correctly targeted because there is good communication between you and your physician. You have the help of both language and nonverbal body language to communicate exactly what you are experiencing. You can clearly articulate in words the quality of the pain to easily guide the doctor to the correct solution.

The decreased ability to communicate becomes a significant barrier for patients with severe dementia and also for the individuals involved with assessing and managing their pain symptoms. (It should be noted that the pain experienced by patients with dementia is not caused by the dementia per se, but instead it is linked with co-morbid conditions that become more prevalent with age such as arthritis, osteoporosis, peripheral neuropathy, heart disease, etc.) This issue of communication is crucial because one of the key tenets of the palliative approach to end-of-life care is to provide relief from pain and other symptoms in order to improve the comfort and quality of life for patients (see page 14, "Why Palliative Care?"). Health care professionals must therefore become reliant on nonverbal or behavioural cues for the detection of different types of pain (e.g., physical, emotional) as well as other symptoms that may cause discomfort, such as trouble breathing or nausea. Some of these cues may include repetitive shouting, sweating, facial expression, and emotional or physical agitation.

It must be noted, however, that while these cues are helpful in providing evidence of the presence of pain, they are unfortunately not as accurate in assessing the intensity of the pain. In some cases, close friends or family members may be able to read the facial expressions of their loved one more accurately than health care professionals, as they are more attuned to their gestures and expressions, and they can then act as a voice for the patient. Yet despite this limitation, health care professionals must try their very best even in the face of difficult communicative challenges to achieve this goal.

A Call for Education

In order to properly address the wide range of issues that are faced by those living with dementia and those responsible for their care, there needs to be not only more public awareness, but also professional awareness. It may be helpful to develop workshops or training seminars, for example, for health care providers and for families to be able to understand the issues involved in achieving the goals of care at this stage of dementia and of life. These would be designed to accompany a set of valid and reliable guidelines and principles that would exemplify the best practice in this area of care. Health care and social service providers would be educated in a practical, insightful, and meaningful way, hopefully through hands-on training and role playing.

Though a guide like this is a good starting point, it would be most useful to create ways to ensure that this information would translate into actual practice. The aim would be for the professionals to be able to leave the workshop better equipped with the knowledge and experience to be able to actively implement this approach in their world of caring.

These ideas could also be incorporated into health care professionals' educational curricula, including not only symptom management but also the psycho-social-cultural dimensions of palliative care for late-stage dementia. It would be important to emphasize an appreciation for cultural and spiritual diversity and how this affects the delivery of care.

From the family or caregiving perspective, there should be learning modules, workshops, online programs, and any other way that health care professionals can be exposed to the principles required for good care to support the family through their loved ones' illness trajectory. These educational and supportive approaches for health care professionals should be information-driven (e.g., learning about the clinical course of dementia, learning about the different types of treatment options, learning about the palliative care approach, etc.). Educational materials and programs for families would include salient information but would focus primarily on being a safe and supportive place to share experiences and challenges that come up in the caregiving process.

Summary

The palliative care approach to late-stage dementia is congruent with the aims of the person-centred approach. Regardless of the degree of impairment, all individuals deserve the promotion of well-being and quality of life. This can be achieved by taking the perspective of the patient, by treating each individual as unique and someone of worth, and finally by creating a supportive social environment. The goal always must be, at all stages of the terminal phase of the illness and in the end-of-life situation, to provide comfort, compassion, and care to the individuals being cared for and their families, who are struggling and confronting what usually is a long and challenging experience.

- In the past few years, there has indeed been an ever-increasing interest in taking a palliative care approach for late-stage dementia.
- The mission now becomes to combine our knowledge of dementia and the palliative care experience that has been gleaned from the treatment of other conditions such as cancer and which may coexist in people experiencing late-stage dementia; and to sufficiently explore the clinical challenges that arise when taking this approach.
- Many of the challenges being faced during the later stages of dementia come down to ethical decisions and considerations, and these should be properly discussed, debated, and explored for all those involved in the process and delivery of care.

AVOIDING AND DEALING WITH FAMILY CONFLICT

Despite Best Efforts

Sometimes conflicts among family members occur, despite all the best efforts by members of the health care team and family members who understand and appreciate the importance of a cooperative and supportive approach to end-of-life care. It is not surprising, even though one might hope and expect family members to have the best interests of their loved ones as the priority. At times, their interpretation of their loved one's wishes may differ from that of other members of the family.

There are a number of ways that people try to avoid conflict occurring among those that love them or that will become party to the end-of-life decisions. Some seniors recognize early on that there is substantial conflict within their circle of potential decision-makers, and they try to take steps to avoid further conflicts. If the possibility of conflict is based on mere ineffectual communication, it might be best dealt with by a family meeting of all the parties. For many families, this is not an easy undertaking, and there may be a great reluctance to broach the subject, either because it is believed to be bad luck to talk about such issues or because it is just an uncomfortable topic.

It is key that everyone concerned should take the necessary steps to avoid potential conflicts even when they all believe that they will have the best intentions and best interests uppermost in their minds when decisions might have to be made. It is not uncommon for family members, especially in the midst of a medical crisis, to revert to basic responses rather than well thought-out or previously communicated wishes or values expressed by their loved one.

Some individuals, in order to avoid health care interventions that they oppose on principle, will create an *advance directive* or "living will." This is especially important to some if they have witnessed, through family or among friends, a situation of late-stage dementia. Witnessing a person's inability to participate in important decisions or care trajectories that contradict one's values can be a powerful motivator. It is for that reason that many individuals choose to undertake an advance directive. This is often done with the assistance of a lawyer and input from a physician with whom you can express your concerns and wishes so that they are translated into useful and meaningful medical conditions about which decisions might have to be made.

The difficulty with such a process is that sometimes the concepts and terminology used may not reflect the realities of future medical practice, which may lead to ambiguities. Also, if the contents and intentions of the document are not discussed with those who are likely to be responsible for its interpretation, it could be that considerable differences in opinion might result.

In order to avoid conflicts in the end-of-life decision-making stage of dementia, use the process of developing an advance directive as an opportunity not only to generate a written record of wishes and values, but more importantly, as an opportunity to have the foundational discussions about beliefs, values, wishes, and preferences. This way, the family member or person who is the substitute decision-maker will be best equipped to interpret the document and make decisions that are not explicitly covered within it.

At times, disagreements continue right through the very last stages of life, and staff members can be faced with conflict and disagreement among family members. If these conflicts cannot be readily resolved by discussion, it may be necessary to bring in help to try to resolve conflicts. Those professionals who can be of help beyond the clinical health care providers may include social workers or ethicists, if the centre has one available or can access one through a cooperative network. The last and least desirable step is to turn to the regulatory and legal system, which can resolve such conflicts, often at great personal and emotional cost to all the parties involved.

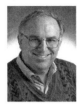

Dr. Gordon Discusses

We were sitting at the table, the two siblings and their spouses. It was a meeting organized by the unit's social worker, who explained to me, "They have come a long way in their discussions, but they are still stuck with the direction that they want to take if the mother becomes ill again with pneumonia. If we do not resolve this issue, we are going to have a difficult time when the next illness occurs."

I had the mother's advanced care directive, which had been written more than ten years previously, when she was clearly mentally capable. The document made sense to me and seemed to be fairly self-evident as to the preferred limitations of treatment. It was drafted by a lawyer, but the details were not discussed with either of the patient's two children.

I explained to the family that in my role as ethicist, I would try to guide them through this challenging decision-making process, and with my understanding of law, ethics, and clinical medicine, I would try and help them reach a consensus on appropriate clinical interventions that would respect her previously expressed wishes. I told them of concerns about "living wills," that they sometimes focus on out-of-date decisions and terminology and rarely provide an overall description of the person's life philosophy and values.

I also said, "At the end of this process, it is important to me, and I believe to your mother, that you will feel sufficiently comfortable that you've served your mother well and reflected and respected her wishes. If this is not the case, you will end up being in conflict with each other, and you may end up becoming what in essence will be life-long enemies because you will believe that the other did a disservice to this person who you both love very much."

I continued, "I am willing to venture that one of the main reasons your mother went to the trouble of writing this document and hiring a lawyer to help her was to prevent conflict between you while also achieving the kind of end-of-life care that she desired. So my goal is to have you agree to a plan of action that will be satisfactory to both of you and in keeping with what you think she would have wanted."

It was a long back and forth process, but after a number of hours of discussion, we arrived at a consensus that seemed to adequately satisfy both siblings in form and in substance. We agreed in principle that whatever care could be provided within the context of the home for the aged would be provided. We discussed with the nurse manager and physician what interventions could be provided without transferring the mother to a general hospital. This alleviated their concern that their mother would end up in the unfamiliar and often technologically driven acute health care system. The physician, in concurrence with the nurse manager, agreed that certain types of interventions, if desired, could be provided. For example, if there were an infection, antibiotics could be provided non-intravenously and any necessary fluids could be provided subcutaneously (under the skin). These measures would be less stressful and easier to administer, and would provide some relief if the mother should need them. This addressed the daughter's concern; she had been asking for more intervention initially. With these provisions, it was agreed that proper care could be provided, and the daughters would not feel that they were not fulfilling the wishes of their mother as they interpreted them.

The mother died some weeks later, and they were all there and in agreement to the limits of care that were provided. And the mother was able to realize her hope for a peaceful death, unmarred by the latest in medical technology.

Summary

- Ideally family members should find ways to communicate with each other so as to avoid conflicts during the difficult end-of-life period.

- Some conflicts occur as part of life-long dysfunction and disagreements among family members.

- In order to try to avoid conflict, it is sometimes worthwhile to elaborate on one's personal wishes and values and to document them in an *advance directive* or "living will" document.

- When there is conflict, it is sometimes necessary to get outside help from skilled individuals who can explain the ethical and legal principles involved in supporting end-of-life decision-making.

Appendix A:
Symptom Management:
Maintaining Comfort

This section drew on information from a number of resources listed in the references.

Managing Symptoms

When discussing the management of symptoms in the latter stages of dementia, it is important to understand the anticipated level of function, participation, and trajectory of the dying process. Some symptoms occur in those with late-stage dementia who are still reasonably mobile and able to participate in some levels of personal and social activities. For them, some interventions would be preferable to others; for example, the use of medications for symptoms whose side effects would be severely detrimental to a still-mobile person. For those in the very late stages of dementia or who, because of other factors, are already primarily bed- or chair-bound and not mobile, other approaches to care might be deemed appropriate that would be considered excessive in those still mobile. Which approach to care to take is a combination of clinical judgment and the wishes of those responsible for clinical decision-making based on previously expressed wishes or the best interests of the person for whom such difficult decisions are being made.

There are many symptoms, both physical and psychological, that are common to patients experiencing end-stage dementia, as well as diseases for which palliative approaches to care may be suitable. Many patients experience multiple symptoms at once or in sequence. Cognitive impairment and difficulties in communicating can make symptom assessment a challenging task, and so unfortunately many symptoms go unrecognized, untreated, or undertreated.

Assessing Symptoms

A word of caution: *These suggestions are general in nature and for reference only. They should not be used to replace the judgments, opinions, and discretion of the caregiver or the opinions of health care professionals. Instead, let this section guide you in the appropriate direction to get further assessments and, where necessary, provide the basis for consideration of interventions.*

The experience of symptoms is subjective, and so the primary source of information, if available, is the patient's self-report. Even if the individual is able to provide verbal communication, many patients are reluctant to report their symptoms because of:

- **Fear:** Patients may be worried about what their symptoms represent, the medications they may be prescribed, or decisions that might be made about their care needs or function.
- **Pride:** Patients may not want to be viewed as "complainers" or be deemed as a person with a disability that might undermine their function or independence.

This is when non-verbal cues such as facial expressions or response to various interventions become especially important.

Symptom assessments should occur at regular intervals following initiation of treatment to follow the effectiveness of the treatment plan, and upon a report of new symptoms.

The following steps can be used a general guide:

1. Identify the possible causes of the symptom.
2. Measure the quality and intensity of the symptom.
3. Recognize and assess the multidimensional aspect of the symptom.
- Physical (including impact on functional ability)
- Psychosocial (psychological distress, use of alcohol and other non-medical drugs, cognitive status, previous history of depression, coping patterns with previous stressors, nature of the family structure and family dynamics)
- Cultural
- Spiritual

There are many assessment tools available, especially for the management of physical discomfort and pain. Refer to Appendix B.

In addition to standard medical interventions that may primarily utilize medications, there are other non-medicinal approaches carried about by social workers, psychologists, massage therapists, non-traditional practitioners, and chaplains, for example.

Prescribed and well-recognized over-the-counter medications are an important component of symptom relief. If symptoms are assessed with care and the issues covered below are followed correctly, medications can often safely provide the desired effect of improving and alleviating symptoms while minimizing the risk of adverse effects.

The Canadian Medical Association has outlined the following principles for medication use in seniors. While these guidelines are intended for the general population, they are also applicable to medication use at the end of life and in those experiencing the latter stages of dementia. The main aspects of the recommendations are:

- **Know the patient:** Be familiar with the specific diagnosis and the symptoms being treated before using medication. Be aware of all the medications that the patient is taking. These include all prescription medication, over-the-counter products, and any herbal, homeopathic, or naturopathic agents. Health care and social service providers should assume that complementary therapies are being used and inquire about them as part of the routine assessment. It is also important to know the history of non-medical drugs, such as alcohol, tobacco, and caffeine. Monitor seniors on a regular basis for the development of adverse drug reactions. In particular, pay attention to cognitive status and be aware of the potential for delirium.
- **Be aware of underlying medical issues:** Thses may prohibit the use of certain classes of medication.
- **Establish treatment goals:** With the patient and his/her family, establish treatment goals for symptom management and determine how achievement of those goals will be established. Regularly assess the adequacy of response and review goals.
- **Know the drugs:** In general, start with low doses and titrate upwards based on response and the emergence of adverse effects. Whenever possible, minimize the number of medications and avoid duplication or complicated dosing regiments to reduce the risk of adverse effects, minimize drug interactions, and improve adherence. Conduct regular medication reviews and discontinue medications if appropriate. If the patient is residing in the community and they or a family caregiver are

responsible for medication administration, verify that they understand the directions for the medication. Encourage the use of compliance aids.

One of the most important barriers to good symptom control is the reluctance to take medication because of fears of addiction, tolerance, or that medications will hasten death. This is particularly true when opioids (sometimes referred to as opiates) are being used. Provide ongoing education about these issues. When appropriate, ask other health care and social providers to assist in education.

- Consider the use of non-pharmacologic therapy: Many non-pharmacologic therapies offered by trained personnel (art therapy, music therapy, occupational therapy, physiotherapy, relaxation techniques, massage therapy, and TENS) can be used along with medications to improve symptoms such as anxiety, generalized weakness, or pain.

Symptom

Depression

What does it look like?

Definition:

- Depression is characterized by at least two weeks of depressed mood or loss of interest accompanied by other symptoms, often referred to as *vegetative symptoms,* such as decreased appetite, abnormal sleep, decreased energy, and loss of enjoyment of ordinary things.
- It can often present itself atypically in older individuals, especially in those with cognitive impairment.
- *Bereavement* is a reaction to the death of a loved one that may produce similar symptoms but is not usually considered to be depression unless the symptoms last longer than two months after the loss.

Affective and behavioural symptoms may occur, such as apathy and lack of enjoyment or pleasure (often referred to as *anhedonia*), often accompanied by social withdrawal. Feelings of sadness, hopelessness, helplessness, guilt, and worthlessness may be present. Somatic (referring to physical or bodily functions) symptoms include agitation/restlessness, anorexia/weight loss, decreased energy, insomnia or hypersomnia, psychomotor retardation, and somnolence. Confusion in someone already suffering from cognitive decline may become exaggerated.

Depression is often associated with co-morbid illness such as dementia or cancer, movement disorders such as Parkinson's, and cardiac and respiratory disorders. Depression can also be aggravated by certain medications, especially sleeping medications and other medications that might affect the mood or levels of consciousness.

Diagnosis can be difficult, as diagnostic criteria (see DSM-IV) rely on neuro-vegetative symptoms that frequently exist without true depression in severe medical illnesses. Seniors often experience bereavement that may be difficult to distinguish from depression. Feelings of guilt and worthlessness may indicate depression rather than bereavement. There is also a need to differentiate sadness appropriate for the illness and the situation from clinical depression.

The following assessment instruments are useful for the senior population:

- If no cognitive impairment is present: Geriatric Depression Scale, Non-verbal Depression Scale, and the Hospital Anxiety and Depression Scale (HADS) can be useful measurement tools. Other instruments for assessment also exist; the important thing is to use whichever validated scales the assessor feels comfortable using.
- If cognitive impairment is present: Cornell Scale for Depression in Dementia.
- Sometimes the most important indicator for a possible diagnosis is the observations of close family members who know the patterns of mood in their loved one.

Suggested approaches and intervention:

Bereavement

- Listen to the individual and encourage him/her to express his/her feelings;
- Assess and offer psychosocial support (additional information about this in following sections).
- Assess and offer bereavement counseling that acknowledges the often multiple losses that may exist, including the losses associated with cognitive decline, if these are acknowledged and understood by the patient, which can depend on the degree of impairment and insight into the illness.

Sadness

- Listen to the individual and encourage him/her to express his/her feelings;
- Be non-judgmental;
- Legitimize the difficulty of the situation;
- Provide reassurances of continued care and interest;

- Respect the person's need to have hope;
- Assess and offer psychosocial support (additional information about this in following sections).

Clinical Depression

- Assess and offer psychosocial support.
- Antidepressant medication:
    - The decision to use antidepressant medication should take into consideration the stage and context of the person and his/her illness.
    - Medication generally takes several weeks to improve mood.
    - Some agents may improve sleep and/or pain control in some individuals.
    - The choice of medication will depend on previous response. If there is a past history of depression, presentation, and side-effect profile, start with low doses and titrate the dose upwards to the necessary response.

Tricyclic antidepressants

- Desipramine or nortriptyline generally have a more favourable side-effect profile. Must beware of hyponatremia and hypotension with nortriptyline.
- Amitriptyline, imipramine, and doxepin exhibit high anticholinergic activity.
- All tricyclics can cause increased confusion in individuals already suffering from cognitive decline and are therefore not the drug class of first choice.
- Initiate at 10 mg orally once daily and titrate upwards by 10–25 mg every 7–14 days.
- Usual maximum daily dose in seniors is 100 mg but may be considerably less in those individuals already suffering from cognitive impairment or severe dementia.
- If individual does not appear to be responding, check serum level or consider changing to another class of antidepressant.

SSRIs (Selective Serotonin Reuptake Inhibitors)

This class of drug has in many instances replaced tricyclics as the class used to treat depression in elderly people, especially in those with some degree of cognitive impairment. There are many SSRIs on the market at this time.

Which medication is chosen is usually based on the experience and preferences of the prescribing physician. In people with cognitive decline or advanced dementia, it is important to consider drugs in which small starting doses are possible (pills that can be split rather than capsules) with very gradual increases in dose, depending on response and tolerance. Physicians must warn patients and families of possibilities of loss of appetite and nausea as possible side effects. It is better to avoid medications with very long half-lives.

It is not possible to list the various SSRIs, as there are new ones on the market all the time with variations in attributes, dosing, and apparent benefit and tolerance.

All SSRIs can exhibit drug interactions; refer to appropriate drug interaction sources.

SNRIs (Serotonin-Norepinephrine Reuptake Inhibitors)

This class of drug is a relatively recent enhancement of the previously mentioned SSRIs. For some people, the medications may also have a beneficial effect in certain types of pain, especially those that come from nerves (so-called neuropathic pain such as one sees in diabetes mellitus). This class of drugs is generally not used along with other antidepressants, and it shares many of the side effects with SSRIs.

When life expectancy is less than six weeks, which means that the dementia has likely been complicated by other co-morbidities, it is sometimes useful to consider treatments with the following agents, which may have an activating effect rather than a true antidepressant effect:

- Ritalin (methylphenidate)
- Alertec (modafinil)
- Decadron (dexamethasone)

Psychomotor retardation/somnolence

- Methylphenidate 2.5 mg by mouth twice daily (before breakfast and lunch to prevent insomnia at night) and titrate to response by 2.5 mg twice daily every other day (usual daily dose may go up to 40 mg but may be less well tolerated in elderly individuals with cognitive decline or dementia).
  - Do not use in those with hyperactive delirium or severe anxiety.

- Can cause confusion and hallucinations in some people, especially those with cognitive impairment; discontinue if this occurs.
- Some clinicians suggest a test dose given in the morning with assessment for adverse central nervous system effects at two hours.
- Avoid late afternoon and evening doses, as the drugs can interfere with sleep.
- Can be useful in the medically ill.
- Rapid but sometimes limited response.
- Avoid in patients with coronary artery disease and arrhythmias.
- Alertec (modafinil) start at 50 mg daily given in the morning and increase gradually up to a dose of 100 mg daily, unless there is no response and no evidence of side effects.

Complementary Therapies

- St. John's Wort: Do not use in conjunction with other antidepressants due to potential drug interactions. This herb may be of some benefit in persons with mild depression. I would be very reluctant to use in people with cognitive impairment or dementia. Dose is 300 mg tid.
- Homeopathy: There is little scientific basis for many treatments in this category, but some people would prefer such interventions rather than standard medications. Patients are often concerned about side effects.

Anxiety

What does it look like?

In the general population, symptoms of anxiety may present in a variety of ways including:

- Agitation or restlessness
- Inability to focus and loss of concentration
- Chest pain or discomfort
- Complaints of heartburn or other non-specific gastrointestinal symptoms
- A choking sensation
- Sensation of shortness of breath or smothering
- Diarrhea
- Dizziness or lightheadedness
- Insomnia
- Sweating, tachycardia, and tremors or shaking
- In later stages of dementia, symptoms may result in increased mental confusion and agitation.

- *How it is caused?*

Anxiety is often a co-morbid disorder associated with psychosocial issues such as lack of family or caregiver support, fear of dying, fear of being a burden to loved ones, and financial concerns. Frequently associated physical conditions include respiratory disease with dyspnea (shortness of breath), cardiovascular disease, chronic pain, delirium, dementia, and depression. It is important to point out that depression sometimes presents itself as anxiety.

Other precipitating factors are medication effects, especially in the terminal phase of illness, including end-stage dementia. Caregivers may also use less benzodiazepines and opioids if there is a decreased level of consciousness leading to withdrawal states, which often present as agitation or anxiety. These symptoms may become clinically evident days later than might be expected in young, healthy adults. Withdrawal causing anxiety and agitation can also occur as the less alert individual reduces alcohol or nicotine consumption.

Suggested approaches and interventions

It is important to provide reassurance and a familiar, safe environment. A psychosocial assessment should be conducted and support provided as appropriate. Spiritual support may be helpful. Non-pharmacological therapies that can be considered include therapeutic touch, relaxation therapy, music therapy and art therapy, massage therapy, and breathing exercises. Such interventions might be particularly useful in those with cognitive impairment as they do not carry with them the problems of medication's side effects. Other interventions are:

- Managing unresolved symptoms, such as pain or dyspnea
- Treating underlying depression if present
- Managing delirium if present
- Managing behavioural symptoms associated with dementia (this may require, among other things, the use of psychoactive medications noted in subsequent sections)
- Considering intermediate acting benzodiazepines such as those noted below if symptoms persist despite other interventions:
  - Lorazepam: initiate 0.25–0.5 mg orally, subcutaneously, sublingually once to twice daily for a short period
  - Oxazepam: initiate 7.5–15 mg orally once to twice daily for a short period (used primarily for sleep and less often in anxiety states)

Note that benzodiazepines can cause paradoxical reactions with increased agitation in some patients. We should generally avoid benzodiazepines with long half-lives for anxiety, as their effect is prolonged in elderly patients. These include:

- Diazepam
- Flurazepam
- Chlordiazepoxide (Although not a benzodiazepine, this drug is on occasion used for anxiety when other medications are ineffective.)

Other drugs not typically used in anxiety but at times useful, effective, and well tolerated:

- SSRIs and SNRIs: This is first choice of the antidepressant medications that can be useful in the treatment of anxiety. Sometimes because of the lag time in effect of an SSRI, a drug such as lorazepam may be required for breakthrough severe anxiety states.
- Antipsychotics: These may also on occasion be useful, as may older antidepressants such as Trazodone.

Complementary therapies can include:

- Acupuncture
- Aromatherapy
- Biofeedback
- Therapeutic touch
- Massage therapy

In individuals with cognitive decline and advanced dementia, benzodiazepines should be avoided if possible or used for short periods. However, benzodiazepines are used specifically for severely disturbing end-of-life symptoms, such as the extreme restlessness known as terminal restlessness.

Weight Loss/Anorexia/Cachexia

What does it look like?

Definitions:

Anorexia is a decreased or total loss of appetite.
Cachexia, otherwise known as "wasting," is malnutrition characterized by

clinically significant weight loss, including both muscle mass and adipose tissue.

The clinical presentation of weight loss and, at its extreme, anorexia and/or cachexia may include:

- Fatigue
- Drowsiness
- Lethargy
- Chronic nausea
- Loss of strength and energy
- Asthenia (generalized weakness)
- Skin breakdown
- Chronic wounds

How it is caused?

The anorexia-cachexia syndrome in the elderly population is associated with many disease processes, including malignancy, cardiac disease, COPD, dementia, delirium, depression, untreated hyperthyroidism, and Parkinson's disease. For those suffering from late-stage cognitive impairment or dementia, there is often a decrease in the desire for and ability to eat normally, including keeping food in the mouth without properly chewing or swallowing. This is often one of the critical events in the trajectory of dementia requiring major decisions by the family in terms of the future approach to care.

Other factors that can cause or contribute to anorexia include dislike of institutional food or ethnic food preferences, oral complications (painful mouth sores, thrush, dry mouth, poorly fitting dentures), dysphagia or odonophagia (painful swallowing), taste disorders, nausea, vomiting, and uncontrolled pain. Caregivers may sometimes not recognize that the senior requires assistance with feeding. Sometimes medications can interfere with the desire for food, and loss of appetite might ensue.

Suggested approaches and interventions

If the problem is altered taste:

- Discontinue suspected medications, if possible.
- Choose foods that address preference for taste and texture.
- Increase seasoning with various and more novel herbs and spices than the person may have preferred in the past.
- Encourage fluid intake.

If the problem is anorexia:

- Identify and treat underlying causes, if appropriate (depression, dementia, delirium, nausea/vomiting).
- Encourage smaller, more frequent meals.
- Be willing to forgo some previously adhered to dietary restrictions (diabetic, low fat, low salt, or other restrictions for chronic disease).
- Encourage individuals to eat when hungry and have food available when it is requested.
- Use a small plate to give the impression of having a complete meal.
- Discontinue or reduce dose of suspected medications, if possible.
- Employ medications to stimulate appetite.

Medications may produce an increase in appetite and small weight gain (mainly fat), but they can also be associated with adverse effects that may limit their use. Evidence in frail seniors is limited, and these medications are recommended only for short-term use when other interventions have failed and individuals find anorexia and its associated weight loss particularly distressing. Individuals and their families should be counseled that while appetite may improve, weight gain may be minimal.

- Dexamethasone: 1–4 mg daily
- Megace (megestrol) acetate: 80 mg–160 mg two or three times daily in gradually increasing doses. It can sometimes have a dramatic effect on the person's desire to eat and food intake.
- Ritalin (methylphenidate)
- Alertec (modafanil)
- Zyprexa (olanzapine)

If the problem has reduced nutritional intake or increased metabolic need (i.e., malignancy):

- Determine if assistance with feeding is required, which occurs quite often in people with late-stage cognitive impairment or dementia.
- Consult a dietician to assess dietary needs and preferences. Identify food preferences and provide these to the individual. Do not be afraid to provide foods that in the past might have been avoided for "health and lifestyle" purposes, as in the late stage of dementia, the long-term prognosis is very limited. Being able to take in and enjoy food becomes an activity of very high importance.
- Meet caloric and protein requirements.

- Use caloric and protein supplements if tolerated. These can be diluted in water or with ice chips.

Medications used to treat anorexia

Drug: **Dexamethasone**

Dose range: 1–4 mg daily, usually in divided doses.
Increase in appetite may last only a few weeks.
May cause or contribute to:

- Hyperglycemia
- Oral candidiasis
- Confusion
- Electrolyte abnormalities
- Myopathy (muscle weakness)
- Increased susceptibility to infection

Drug: **Megestrol acetate**

Dose range: Dosages of 160–480 mg per day found to increase appetite in persons with cancer, but no significant weight gain.
Dosages of 400 mg daily in residents of a long-term care facility with a wide range of conditions including dementia have been found to improve appetite but may be associated with adverse effects that limit use. Starting dose is usually 80 mg per day to avoid nausea: may increase risk of clotting.
May cause or contribute to:

- Hyperglycemia
- Edema
- Confusion
- Thrombo-embolic complications (i.e., DVT, PE)
- Vaginal bleeding upon withdrawal

If there is no benefit from megestrol, try:

- Ritalin
- Modafinil
- Olanzapine

Complementary Therapies:

- Acupuncture
- Therapeutic touch
- Traditional Chinese medicine

Constipation

In most ordinary individuals, even those with a number of chronic diseases, constipation may be an uncomfortable nuisance. In those suffering from end-stage dementia, the lack of adequate bowel movements, severe constipation, or bowel impaction can result in significant discomfort and serious agitation. This may be erroneously attributed to their cognitive state, resulting in the use of medications to deal with agitation, which inadvertently can aggravate the constipation and may at the extreme lead to obstipation (very severe constipation often leading to bowel obstruction), bowel obstruction, and even death.

What does it look like?

Acute constipation means there has been no or inadequate bowel movement for three or more days.

Chronic constipation involves problems with bowel movements that are recurrent or a constant problem or that last over a prolonged period of time. Some of the signs and symptoms of constipation include a reduced number or no bowel movements with increased stool consistency (hardness), flatulence, bloating, or a feeling of incomplete evacuation following a bowel movement.

Sometimes constipation can also present as overflow diarrhea in the presence of fecal impaction. It may be associated with anorexia, nausea and vomiting, and confusion. The danger when this occurs is that treatment may erroneously be focused on the loose bowel movements and treatments provided that will decrease the loose bowel movements, thereby aggravating the constipation or even transform it into a bowel obstruction.

How it is caused?

Constipation can have various causes or precipitating or aggravating factors:

- Confusion
- Immobility

- Poor dietary intake
- Poor fluid intake
- Weakness
- Related to malignancy:
  - Post-operative states especially following bowel surgery
  - Intestinal obstruction
  - Spinal cord compression
  - Hypercalcemia

Concurrent disease states

- Hypothyroidism
- Hypokalemia
- Diabetes
- Diverticular disease

Anal/rectal pathology

- Hemorrhoids
- Anal fissure/stenosis
- Superficial ulcerations

Medications

- Opioids
- Iron
- Medications with anticholinergic effects
  - Tricyclic antidepressants
  - Neuroleptic medications
  - Some calcium preparations/supplements in some individuals
  - Medications used in urinary bladder hyperactivity
  - Medications that are not primarily anticholinergic in action but have anticholinergic effects. It may be necessary to review medication side effects from reliable resources to confirm such pharmacological activities.
- Be especially vigilant when over-the-counter medications are taken, as some used in cold and flu preparations have ingredients that have anticholinergic effects.

Medications and preparations that may be causing or aggravating constipation should be discontinued if possible. A dietary history should be taken to assure it contains good fibre content and adequate fluid intake. One cereal combination that has been quite effective from long-standing clinical observation is a mixture of oatmeal and a product known as Red River Cereal, which contains flax as well as other ingredients. This combination, especially when served with fruit or prunes instead of sugar, can be a very effective promoter of more normal bowel movements.

Bulk-forming agents

Psyllium

- Can be used in chronic constipation if non-pharmacologic interventions do not produce results.
- Administer with meals and avoid bedtime administration.
- Must be given with abundant fluids.
- Must be given on a regular basis (not p.m.).
- Avoid if individuals receive opioids or other constipating medications that alter gut peristalsis; fluid intake is less than 1000 ml per day; there is a suspected impaction, ileus, or bowel obstruction; or the individual is at risk of aspiration.

Stool softeners

Docusate Calcium: capsule stool softener
Dosage: 240–480 mg/day

- Use in the short-term to avoid straining.
- The value of chronic use is unproven.
- High doses may cause anal leakage and excoriation of perianal tissue.

Docusate Sodium: liquid stool softener
Dosage: 200–400 mg/day

- Medicine is concentrated and has a very bitter taste. Dilute in juice if given by mouth. Dilution is not required if administered by tube feed, such as a PEG tube.
- Calcium and sodium content of preparations are clinically insignificant.

Mineral Oil: available in liquid or gel
Dosage: 30 ml as required

- Use in the short-term for excessively hard stool or as initial treatment for impaction. Following up with milk of magnesia and/or an enema may be required.
- Avoid long-term use.
- Avoid administering to individuals at risk of aspirations (liquid or gel products).
- Long-term use may cause anal leakage and excoriation of perianal tissue.
- Long-term use may reduce absorption of fat-soluble vitamins (i.e., vitamins A, D and E).

Saline agents

Magnesium hydroxide (MOM): liquid or tablets
Dosage: Usual dosage is 15–30 ml or 4–8 tablets at bedtime. Larger dosages of 45–90 ml may be required for refractory, chronic constipation

- Suitable for chronic use
- May be administered regularly or on a prn basis
- Avoid in individuals with renal failure due to high magnesium content
  - Liquid: 41 mmol per 30 ml
  - Tablet: 5.3 mmol

Sodium phosphates
Dosage: Dose for fecal impaction, 45 ml initially; may repeat in five hours if necessary. Dilute in 120 ml of sweet juice. Follow by 240 ml of juice.

- Useful for management of fecal impaction
- Extremely salty taste requires liberal dilution as described in dosage section
- High sodium content: 434 mmol/90 ml (equivalent to 3 L normal saline)
- Due to high sodium content, avoid with individuals requiring sodium restriction or those with congestive heart failure.

PEG-lyte (powder containing polyethehylene glycol 3350 NaSO4, NaH3O2, NaCl, KCl)

Dosage: For fecal impaction, administer 100–150 ml by mouth, NG tube, or gastrostomy tube every 30 minutes (i.e., 1–2 L over 3–4 hours). Repeat next day if necessary. If this dosage rate is not tolerated, give smaller volumes less frequently.

- Use for fecal impaction
- Dosage rate is often not tolerated if individual is very ill and/or frail
- Negligible absorption of electrolytes
- Very salty taste

Lax-a-day, MiraLAX, and RestoraLAX are new formulations of polyethylene glycol that can be bought over the counter as a powder to be taken with liquid dilutant (such as water or juice) to be used short-term or on an occasional basis.

The bottle top is a measuring cap marked to contain 17 grams of the powder (about 1 heaping tablespoon). Dissolve the powder in 8 ounces (1 cup) of water and drink. It is best to take the mixture first thing in the morning. It can be taken on either an empty or full stomach.

Stimulating agents

In general, these provide direct stimulation of intestinal smooth muscle activity and enhance secretion of water and electrolytes into bowel lumen.

- They are used to manage acute constipation if bowel obstruction is ruled out.
- These are the first choice in the prevention and management of opioid-induced constipation and can be used in conjunction with other agents for this purpose.
- Some individuals may complain of abdominal cramping. Decrease dose or switch to another stimulant agent.
- Stimulating agents are contraindicated in bowel obstruction.

Cascara Sagrada: available as 300 mg tablet or fluid extract
Dosage: Usual dose for tablet is 300–600 mg at bedtime. Usual dose for fluid extract is 5–10 ml at bedtime.

MOM + Cascara: concentrated liquid, 15 ml is equivalent to 30 ml MOM + 5 ml cascara

Dosage: Usual dose is 15 ml at bedtime

Bisacodyl tablets
Dosage: Usual dose is 5–10 mg at bedtime
Bisacodyl tablet is enteric-coated; avoid administration with MOM or antacids.

Senna: Available as senna tea. Many people, especially those from overseas, may use senna-containing tea on a habitual basis for their bowels not realizing that it has pharmacological properties. For those who have used such products all their lives, there may be a problem with chronic overuse, which may be one of the causes of chronic constipation and the need for habitual use of stimulating agents.
Dosage: Usual dose is 2–4 tablets at bedtime

Osmotic agents

Lactulose
Dosage: Usual dose 15–30 ml daily
May be effective in those individuals who have not responded to other laxatives.

Sorbital
Dosage: Usual dose 15–30 ml daily

- Very sweet taste. Can be diluted in juice or warm milk
- May cause some bloating and gas pains

Suppositories

Glycerin

- Works by a combination of local stimulation of the anus and lubrication of the outflow tract in those with very hard stools and painful expulsion.
- Use glycerin suppository first, then bisacodyl suppository if glycerin fails.

Bisacodyl
Dosage: 10 mg

- Chronic, routine use may cause irritation of rectal mucosa
- Stimulates the anus

Enemas

Do rectal exams first to ensure no impaction

Sodium Phosphate

- Enema should be prewarmed in tap water
- Requires retention of fluid until stool evacuation
- Use proper administration to avoid abrasion of rectal wall
- May repeat dose in 30 minutes if necessary
- Frequent use may damage rectal mucosa

Mineral Oil Enema

- Enema should be prewarmed in tap water
- Lubricates hard stool in the rectum
- May follow in several hours with other measures

General Principles

- Establish the individual's normal bowel routine:
  - Number of bowel movements per week
  - Consistency, colour, and volume of stool
- Encourage mobilization as tolerated
- Ensure adequate hydration
- Establish a regular toileting routine, as strongest peristalsis occurs in early morning after breakfast
- Sit individual upright when toileting, if tolerated
- Provide as much privacy as possible
- Maintain good perianal care
- Determine adherence with laxative regimen. Patient dislike is a common cause of noncompliance (e.g., taste, abdominal cramping)

If the problem is possible fecal impaction:

- Consider flat plate X-ray of the abdomen to determine the extent of the constipation.

- Use a digital rectal exam to determine presence, amount, and consistency of stool, may then try a glycerin suppository; sodium phosphate enema if suppository not effective in 30 minutes or mineral oil enema if stool is very hard.
  - If there is impaction: try manual disimpaction by a trained health care professional in order to avoid bowel obstruction.
  - Use sodium phosphate oral solution 45 ml po but remember it has a high sodium content—therefore, do not use if sodium restriction, congestive heart failure, or congenital megacolon.
  - PEG-lyte lavage if unable to tolerate sodium load of sodium phosphate oral: 100 ml q 30 minutes or a smaller volumes less frequently if unable to tolerate dosing rate.
  - If impaction in proximal colon, consider tap water enema.

If the problem is prevention of opioid-induced constipation:

- Begin stimulant laxative when opioid initiated—Senna.
- If stool consistency is very hard, add stool softener to reduce straining.
- Administer prune juice, if tolerated.
- Avoid bulk laxatives.
- Consider prokinetic agents, such as domperidone and metoclopramide.
- Methylnaltrexone (Relistor) is a relatively new agent specifically directed towards opioid-induced constipation. It is given by SC injection and may be very effective, especially in those people for whom enemas may be technically difficult and/or very traumatic. Do not use if suspected bowel obstruction.

Nausea/Vomiting

What does it look like?

Nausea in patients can occur with or without vomiting, and in some cases, nausea can be even more distressing to those in the latter situation. Likewise, vomiting may be present without the preceding nausea. In this case, caregivers can probably suspect a mechanical obstruction or decreased intestinal tract motility, particularly if the vomiting occurs soon after eating.

In the case of a suspected mechanical obstruction, there should first be a clinical evaluation ruling out non-malignant causes, such as pseudo-obstruction secondary to fecal impaction or adhesions. One is usually suspicious, as there is often a good deal of bloating of the abdomen accompanied by discomfort. This kind of non-malignant obstruction predominantly occurs in people with pelvic or abdominal disease. There may be a complete obstruction if there are symptoms present such as a large-volume vomit, nausea becoming worse prior to vomiting, nausea becoming relieved after emesis, a colicky-type abdominal pain, and no stool in the rectum when it is examined, as well as minimal, distant, or high-pitched bowel sounds when the abdomen is examined with a stethoscope.

How it is caused?

There are a number of causes for the unpleasant experience of nausea, which can be grouped into four general categories: visceral disturbances, chemical disorders, vestibular disturbances, and central nervous system disturbances.

Visceral Disturbance: Decreased gastrointestinal motility, slow gastric emptying, gastric stasis, ileus; sometimes following abdominal or other surgery
Medications: anticholinergic agents, opioids
Mechanical obstruction due to non-malignant or malignant causes:

- Upper GI tract: malignancies causing gastric outlet obstruction
- Lower GI tract: malignancies (e.g., colon cancer; pelvic cancers such as ovarian cancer)
- Fecal impaction

Mucosal irritation (esophageal or gastric) can come from infections such as esophageal candidiasis or medications such as ASA and NSAIDs (most common) as well as acid reflux. At the extreme, there may be an associated gastrointestinal bleeding from the stomach, duodenum, or esophagus.

Chemical Disorders
Medications: Some medications may cause nausea or vomiting through their effect on the chemoreceptor trigger zone. These include opioids for pain, chemotherapy, and radiation therapy. Many commonly used medications have nausea listed as a possible adverse effect; if unsure, all medications should be considered as a possible factor in the cause of this symptom.

Biochemical disorders: Hypercalcemia may occur in malignant conditions such as myeloma, breast, and lung cancers. Electrolyte disturbances may be precipitated by medications such as diuretics or by disease such as kidney or liver failure.

Vestibular Disturbances

Some medications can affect the function of the inner ear and cause damage to the balance mechanism; such may occur with opioids and certain antibiotics. CNS tumors and metastatic tumors can affect the inner ear or the vestibule-cochlear nerve, especially if they occur at the base of the skull.

Central Nervous System Disturbances

These include elevated intracranial pressure and skull base fractures.

Psychological and emotional factors

Some individuals manifest stress and anxiety through physical symptoms including nausea and vomiting.

Suggested approaches and interventions

The following categories are classes of medications used to treat nausea and vomiting, along with their sites of action.

1. Antihistamines

- Meclizine: vestibular centre, vomiting centre
- Cyclizine: vestibular centre, vomiting centre
- Dimenhydrinate: vestibular centre, vomiting centre

2. Butyrophenones

Haloperidol: chemoreceptor trigger zone

3. Phenothiazines

- Prochlorperazine: chemoreceptor trigger zone
- Methotrimeprazine: vomiting centre, chemoreceptor trigger zone

4. Atypical Antipsychotics

- Olanzapine
- Risperidone (less commonly used for this purpose)

5. Anticholinergic agents

- Hyoscine butylbromide: reduces gut motility (bowel paralysis), reduces gastric secretions
- Scopolamine: vomiting centre, reduces gut motility

6. Prokinetic agents

- Domperidone: local gastric prokinetic (enhances gut motility, but works only for poor gastric emptying)
- Metoclopramide: chemoreceptor trigger zone, enhances gut motility

7. Other agents

- Octreotide: reduces colonic secretions
- H2 antagonists (Zantac) or Proton Pump Inhibitors (Prevacid: decrease gastric secretions

8. Cannabinoids

- Nabilone: may cause confusion in the elderly, especially in those with cognitive impairment or dementia

Non-pharmacologic approaches to nausea and vomiting include reducing or eliminating specific triggers such as odours or foods, keeping the room cool, not pressuring the patient to eat, and offering foods and drinks like dry toast, crackers, and flat ginger ale. This may present special problems in individuals suffering from dementia, as it may not be possible to differentiate some of the triggering mechanisms. Sometimes trial and error is necessary to determine if these non-pharmacologic measures might be useful.

If the patient has indeed vomited, it is important to provide good mouth care to clear the taste of emesis. Offer water, dilute juice, or dilute mouthwash to help remove the offending taste and smell that may follow vomiting.

Delirium

What does it look like?

People with dementia are at very high risk of developing delirium. It is an abrupt and severe decline in the ability to focus, sustain, or shift attention. There is an accompanying change in cognition and/or the development of a perceptual disturbance that isn't accounted for by dementia alone. It develops over a brief period of time and fluctuates over the duration of the day.

It may present itself as disorientation, agitation/restlessness, or a decreased and/or fluctuating level of consciousness. There could be incoherent speech or rambling with an inability to name objects or to write. Perceptual disturbances such as hallucinations, illusions, and misinterpretations of external stimuli may also occur. A reversal of the sleep-wake cycle is also quite common.

How it is caused?

Delirium is most often multifactorial with a high association of occurrence in those suffering from dementia, especially in the later stages of the disorder. In some individuals with cognitive impairment that has not yet been recognized as such, it is an episode of delirium during a hospitalization or as the result of an infection or new medication that is the first indication to others that the person suffers from cognitive impairment or mild or moderate dementia. It can be caused by:

- Medications (e.g., anticholineric agents, benzodiazepines, narcotics)
- Metabolic disturbances (e.g., hyper and hyponatremia, hypercalcemia, azotemia)
- Infections of any type, bacterial or viral, but especially of the urinary and pulmonary tract
- Depression, sometimes during a serious exacerbation of it or when medications for its treatment are implemented or the dose is increased or changed
- Elevated intracranial pressure secondary to tumor or intracranial bleed, unusual as an event accompanying dementia
- Subdural hematoma, sometimes in individuals with dementia who have recently fallen, especially if they are taking any kind of anticoagulant or platelet inhibitor
- Environmental changes, even the change from day to night, especially in unfamiliar surroundings
- Constipation/fecal impaction, especially when the patient may be relatively immobile, have a limited diet in terms of fibre content, and be without the ability to explain that they have not had a good bowel movement
- Urinary retention

Suggested approaches and interventions

The first approach must always be to remove or address the precipitating event or cause of the delirium whenever possible. Once that is done, other interventions might be of value.

If the problem is:

Agitation/restlessness

Neuroleptics

- Choice of agent depends on side-effect profile and experience
- Initiate therapy at lowest possible dose and increase if necessary
- Dose around the clock until under control, then decrease dose by 25 percent and see if the patient can be gradually weaned off the drug as the underlying condition is brought under control (i.e., the infection is treated, the metabolic disorder resolved)
- Haloperidol 0.5–1.5 mg po or sc q 4–8h (po and sc doses are equivalent)
- Methotrimeprazine (Nozinan) 2.5–5 mg. Q 8–12h po or sc
- Risperidone 0.5–1 mg po bid, sublingual formulation also available
- Olanzapine 2.5–15 mg po daily (SL available)
- Quetiapine 12.5–50 mg, po daily

There needs to be a provision for breakthrough or rescue dosing when these medications are used and the condition is serious.

Benzodiazepines

- Add when there is severe agitation and poor response to optimal doses of neuroleptics
- Lorazepam 0.5–2 mg po or sublingual or sc q 4–6 h pm

Hallucinations/perceptual disturbances
- Reassure individual
- Medications: Same medications that are used in agitation and restlessness (above)

Hallucinations secondary to anti-Parkinsonian agents frequently occur in advanced stages of Parkinson's disease, especially in individuals who also have cognitive impairment. Discontinue (or decrease doses) medications in the following sequence:

1. Anticholinergics
2. Amantadine
3. Dopamine agonists

4. Decrease dose of levodopa preparations, which can result in re-emergence of Parkinsonian symptoms

If inadequate response or re-emergence of severe Parkinsonian symptoms occurs, consider:
- Quetiapine: 12.5–50 mg po daily
- Olanzapine: Initiate at 2.5 mg qhs and gradually increase dose to response (maximum of 15 mg per day). It has some D2 receptor blocking properties, with a potential to worsen Parkinsonian symptoms. Somnolence can be dose limiting.
- Clozapine: initiate at 12.5 mg qhs and gradually increase to 25–75 mg/ day. It can cause agranulocytosis; use weekly CBC with differential to monitor. It can also cause orthostatic hypotension.

Try to identify and manage the underlying cause or contributing factors to hallucinations whenever it is possible to do so. Discontinue medications suspected of causing or contributing to the problem, or at the very least, decrease the dose or switch to a similar type of medication. Provide a safe, familiar, and comfortable environment to decrease the risk of falls, and frequently reorient and reassure the individual. If possible, have a family member or caregiver sit quietly with the individual and speak quietly to them while holding their hand and reassuring them. Some complementary therapies to try are: homeopathy, aromatherapy, massage therapy, music therapy, and therapeutic touch.

Dyspnea/Breathlessness/Respiratory Problems

What does it look like?

Dyspnea is defined as laboured breathing accompanied by a sense of shortness of breath or suffocation. It may be accompanied by a feeling of being smothered or suffocated, anxiety, and difficulty in clearing secretions. Signs may include increased respiratory rate (tachypnea); bronchospasm, which can be identified by the patient's wheezing; use of accessory muscles and intercostal muscles; in-drawing paradoxical breathing; and cyanosis if patient hypoxic. However, individuals may have minimal objective signs but still experience severe shortness of breath. Verbal categorical (none, mild, moderate, severe) or visual analogue scale may be useful to assess the severity of a patient's distress.

How it is caused?

Like delirium, dyspnea/breathlessness/respiratory problems are frequently multifactorial in terms of their causes. These problems may be caused by:

- Cardiac disease, such as congestive heart failure with pulmonary edema
- Respiratory disease
  - Chronic obstructive pulmonary disease
  - Pneumonia of the aspiration type, due to problems with swallowing. Probably the most common type of pneumonia, although viral and secondary bacterial pneumonia are also common, due to increased susceptibility to infection
  - Pneumothorax
  - Pulmonary embolism, especially for patients immobilized and bed-bound
  - Pulmonary fibrosis
  - Tumours (primary or secondary)
- Severe anemia
- Weakness/myopathy

Suggested approaches and interventions

Place the individual in Fowler's Position (semi-sitting position), and use environmental modifications to ease symptoms. Eliminate or reduce environmental irritants (cigarette smoke, perfumes, scents, etc.). Keep the room at comfortable temperature for the individual, and ensure adequate ventilation by using fans, opening windows (avoid excessive cooling), and keeping a clear visual path between the individual and the fan or open window. Relaxation therapy and therapeutic touch can be helpful for anxiety, as can complementary therapies such as acupuncture and aromatherapy.

If the problem is:

- Bronchospasm
  - Salbutamol: 2–3 puffs q 4–8h (with aerochamber) or 2.5–5.0 mg diluted to 3–4 ml with saline q 4–8h via nebulizer
  - Can add ipratropium bromide 2–3 puffs (with aerochamber) or 250–500 ug (can mix with salbutamol) q 4–8h via nebulizer
  - Steroids
    - Prednisone 10-50 mg po once daily or as an inhaler
    - Solumedrol IV
    - Decadron sc
- Cough: This can cause a great deal of discomfort and agitation in individuals with late-stage dementia, as at times there does not seem to be any respite from it. When accompanied by tenacious sputum, it can cause a great deal of discomfort and agitation.

- Cough suppressants
  - Dextromethorphan 15–45 mg po q 4h prn
  - Codeine 10–15 mg po or 5–7.5 mg sc q 4h prn
  - Hydrocodone 2.5–5 mg po q 4–6h prn
  - Morphine 2.5–5 mg po or 1–2.5 mg sc q 4h prn (remember to avoid morphine when there is renal insufficiency or failure; prefer to use hydromorphone or oxycodone; hydromorphone is the first choice, plus no SC alternative for oxycodone
  - Cough assist device to help clear sputum
  - Chest physiotherapy to help clear sputum

- Hypoxia
  - Oxygen saturation less than 90 percent
    - Monitor O_2 saturation to assess ongoing need for oxygen
    - Use cautiously in severe COPD
    - Low-flow O_2 by nasal prongs may be useful
    - In CO_2 retainers, keep O_2 saturation between 88–92 percent

- Malignant Obstruction
  - Steroids
    - Dexamethasone 8–32 mg/day: BID to TID
    - Try to avoid evening dosing to prevent insomnia

- Pleural effusion
  - Thoracentesis
  - If recurrent, use talc or doxycyline pleurodesis, or insert a drainage catheter (for example, a Tenchkoff ™ catheter)

- Pulmonary edema
  - Furosemide 20–120 mg po pm (can give SC—max 20 mg = 2 ml per site)
  - Appropriate cardiac medications
  - Salt and fluid restrictions

- Sensation of breathlessness/smothering/respiratory distress
  - If opioid naïve, morphine 2.5–5 mg po q 2–4h prn or 1–2.5 mg sc q 1–4 h prn (avoid in renal insufficiency or failure; prefer to use hydromorphone or oxycodone)

- If taking opioids, increase dose of same opioid by 25–50% q 4h or add breakthrough doses to given in 24 hours to the previous standing dose given in same 24-hr period total dose
- If severe distress, administer opioids via SC route and consider continuous subcutaneous infusion of opioid
- To manage anxiety:
  - Initiate chlorpromazine at 10–25 mg po q 8–12h
  - Benzodiazepines may be useful in acute distress
    - Lorazepam 0.25–0.5 mg po or sl or sc q 1h prn
    - Midazolam as a subcutaneous infusion may be required in those with severe agitation or restlessness that does not respond to other measures
- Changes in respiration (i.e., Cheyne-Stokes breathing) during last hours of life can be distressful to family members. Provide support and reassurance, and continue pharmacologic management for breathlessness.
- Secretions
  - Use cool mist vaporizer to increase humidity in room (clean daily)
  - Consult physiotherapy to help clear secretions
  - Administer nebulized saline to loosen thick secretions
  - To reduce secretions, provide good mouth care and keep mucous membranes moist, and ensure adequate hydration
    - Glycopyrrolate 0.1–0.4 mg sc tid-qid prn
    - Hyoscine hydrobromide 0.2–0.6 mg sc q 4–6h prn (more sedating than glycopyrrolate)
    - Atropine 0.3–0.6 mg sc q 4h prn
    - Scopolamine patch, 1.5 mg transdermal behind alternating ears q 72h (8–12 hr onset of action)
  - Avoid oropharyngeal/nasopharyngeal suctioning unless absolutely necessary

Noisy secretions during the last few hours of life can be very distressing to family as they are often perceived as discomfort. Provide support and reassurance, and continue pharmacologic management for secretions.

Dysphagia/Oral Complications

What does it look like?

Dysphagia is defined as difficulty swallowing. Oral complications refer to oral/esophageal infections, oral ulcers, and dry mouth. Such complications can occur when there is generalized weakness, following a stroke or when a tumour exists.

Symptoms associated with swallowing difficulty include coughing after taking fluids or food, which may indicate aspiration; a "wet voice" during or after eating; and choking episodes. There may be complaints of sore mouth, painful swallowing, and chest pain or "heartburn," especially after taking fluids or food. Decreased intake of fluids and/or food may result in weight loss. Sometime aspiration can be "silent"—the person and/or caregivers may not be aware of its occurrence until an infection occurs, causing aspiration pneumonia. In individuals with late-stage dementia, this is one of the many events that may be life-threatening or life-ending, depending on how it is addressed, with aggressive treatment or in a palliative comfort-care approach. It is important to avoid the use of straws when drinking fluids in such situations. Use spoons instead, and use sponges for fluid administration to avoid possible abrasions of the mouth caused by a straw.

How it is caused?

Associated specific diseases include cerebrovascular accidents, CNS malignancy, dementia, Parkinson's disease, neuromuscular disorders (myasthenia gravis), multiple sclerosis, and amyotrophic lateral sclerosis (progressive muscular atrophy). In those suffering from late-stage dementia, eating skills are often lost, and food and oral secretions may be kept in the mouth for prolonged periods, which may increase the likelihood of aspiration and local lesions in the mouth. It is often difficult to provide good mouth care to people with late-stage dementia, as often the person does not or cannot cooperate with those providing the care or follow the instructions necessary to provide it. Painful swallowing can follow acid reflux, oral/esophageal candidiasis, radiation treatment to head and neck, and esophageal obstruction. Weakness or sedation and poorly fitting dentures also contribute.

Medications that can affect swallowing are:
- Oral phase of swallowing
  - Dry mouth
    - Anticholinergics
    - Agents with anticholinergic activity (e.g., tricyclic antidepressants, phenothiazines, opioids, some anti-emetics), which are sometimes used in individuals suffering from late-stage dementia
  - Oral lesions
    - Antineoplastics (e.g., 5-fluorouracil)

- Corticosteroids
- Parkinsonian symptoms
  - Neuroleptics
  - Metoclopromide
- Sedation
  - Benzodiazepines
  - Tricyclic antidepressants
  - Phenothiazines
  - Opioids
- Pharyngeal phase of swallowing
  - Parkinsonian symptoms, which may accompany some causes of late-stage dementia, such as Lewy Body dementia or the dementia of late-stage Parkinson's disease
    - Neuroleptics
    - Metoclopramide
- Esophageal phase of swallowing
  - Direct esophageal injury
    - Tetracycline
    - Doxycycline
    - Corticosteroids
    - Potassium salts
    - Biphosphanates used in those with osteoporosis (Many would say that those suffering from late-stage dementia should not be provided with this class of medication because of the risk to esophageal ulceration if not used properly, which may not be possible in those with late-stage dementia. Most important is the fact that the benefits of this class of medication are long-term and not likely to be of much clinical value in this particular population because of the limited life expectancy.)
  - Decreased pressure in lower esophageal sphincter (causing reflux)
    - Anticholinergics and medications with anticholinergic activity
    - Some calcium channel blockers (e.g., dihydropyridines)
    - Nitrates

Suggested approaches and interventions

If the problem is:

- Acid reflux, which can cause painful swallowing
  - To neutralize excess acid
    - Aluminum- and/or magnesium-containing antacids

- 15–30 mls po or q 2h prn
  - Alginic acid
    - or 2–4 chewable tablets po qid pc and hs
- To reduce acid production
  - H2-antagonists
    - Ranitidine 150 mg po qhs to bid (may need to adjust in renal impairment)
    - Famotidine 20–40 mg po daily
    - Cimetidine 300 mg bid (This medication should be avoided in those suffering from late-stage dementia, as it can aggravate confusion and delirium.)
- Proton pump inhibitors
  - Omeprazole 20–40 mg po daily (do not crush tablets)
  - Lansoprazole 15–30 mg po daily
  - Pantoprazole 40 mg daily; enteric-coated, do not crush
- Increase pressure in lower esophageal sphincter, thereby decreasing acid reflux
  - Prokinetic Agents
    - Domperidone 10–20 mg po qid ½ hr ac and hs
    - Metoclopramide 5–10 mg po qid ½ hr ac and hs or 5 mg sc qid ½ hr ac and hs (can go to maximum 20mg qid); may cause EPS with long-term use

- Esophageal ulcers
  - To provide a protective coating over open ulcers
    - Sucralfate 1 gm qid qid sc and hs (It comes in a tablet and oral suspension. The tablet can be crushed, which may be necessary in use for some individuals with late-stage dementia who cannot swallow the tablet.)

- Oral candidiasis
  - Treat infection
    - Nystatin 500,000 units qid po swish and swallow × 14 days. This may be very difficult to accomplish in individuals with late-stage dementia, as the instructions are quite complicated. It can be frozen into popsicle for more palatable administration.
    - Ketoconazole 200 mg po daily to bid × 14 days (200–400mg as single daily dose)

- Itraconazole 100 mg po daily × 14 days
  - Ketoconazole and itraconazole require acidic environment for adequate absorption
  - Concurrent use with H2-antagonist/proton pump inhibitor can result in treatment failure
  - If achlorhydria is suspected, administer with cola beverage to provide sufficient acid absorption
- Fluconazole 100 mg daily ×14 days; decrease dose if estimated creatinine clearance <50 ml/min
- Persons with chronic oral candidiasis require longer treatment period (e.g., 6–12 months)
- Azole antifungals (ketoconazole, itraconazole, fluconazole) can inhibit the metabolism of several medications that may be given concurrently; refer to appropriate drug interactions references.

- Esophageal candidiasis
  - Ketocozole 400 mg po daily × 4–6 weeks
  - Itraconazole 100 mg po daily × 4–6 weeks
  - Fluconazole 100–200 mg po daily × 4–6 weeks

- Mouth care/hygiene: This is especially important in individuals with late-stage dementia, as they may not be able to participate in their own mouth or dental hygiene. Failure to provide good care can result in deterioration in dentition very rapidly and a persistent terrible taste or infections around the teeth that cannot be readily treated once established (periodontitis).
  - Brush teeth and gums regularly with soft brush and fluoride toothpaste or gel. If the person is in his or her last hours of life, apply baking soda mouthwash and medications with sponge swabs.
  - If there is gingivitis or the beginnings of periodontitis, brush with chlorhexidene mouthwash
  - Soak dentures in water with 1 squirt of chlorhexadine soap qhs × 30 days

- Difficulty taking oral fluids and food
  - Consult speech pathologist if there is difficulty swallowing
  - Identify appropriate feeding techniques: positioning, compensatory techniques, appropriate utensils
  - Identify most appropriate consistency
    - Liquids (thin, thick, gelled), solids (minced, pureed)

- Consider palatability as well as ease of chewing, swallowing
  - Education and training for senior, family and caregivers regarding nature of swallowing difficulty and strategies to reduce risk
  - Medications to treat underlying disorders if appropriate

- Dry mouth: See dehydration

- Aphthous ulcers
  - Saline mouth rinse, swish, and spit qid
  - Avoid acidic foods and fluids
  - Use protective dental pastes
    - Steroid containing
      - Dab on oral lesions tid to produce a thin film
      - May decrease pain and shorten duration of episode
    - Non-steroid containing
      - Dab on oral lesion tid pc and hs to produce a thin film
  - Lidocaine viscous 2%
    - Dab on oral lesion tid pc and hs
    - For extensive oral lesions, 15 ml swish and spit or swish and swallow qid
    - No food or fluids within 60 minutes of ingestion, as it may interfere with pharyngeal phase of swallowing

- Excessive salivation
  - Scopolamine 1.5 mg transdermal patch behind alternating ears q 3 days (8–12 hours for effect to begin)
  - Nortriptyline or desipramine 10–25 mg po daily
  - Glycopyrrolate initiate at 1 mg tid
  - Atropine eye drops 1–2 drops in mouth
  - All of these medications can cause vision problems and urinary retention in some individuals because of their anticholinergic properties.

Skin Breakdown/Chronic Wounds

What does it look like?

Pressure sores (also known as bedsores and decubitus ulcers) are caused by prolonged pressure on an area of the skin. These can occur in individuals with end-stage dementia because of decreased mobility in bed or in chairs.

Care must be taken to avoid excessive periods of immobility in order to avoid such occurrences.

A fungating lesion is a tumour that can be observed at the skin surface that may break through the skin and cause ulceration. This would only occur in a person suffering from end-stage dementia if other conditions coexisted with their dementia.

Please note that the staging system presented below does not represent a continuum of progressive damage. For example, stage 1 wounds do not have to progress through each stage to become a stage 4 wound, and a stage 2 wound is more severe than a stage 1 wound.

Stage 1:
- Non-blanchable erythema of intact skin, not to be confused with reactive hyperemia
- May be difficult to identify in individuals whose skin is darkly pigmented or discoloured. In these individuals, warmth, edema, induration (swelling of skin), or hardness may be used as indicators

Stage 2:
- Partial-thickness skin loss involving epidermis and/or dermis
- Superficial ulcer presents as abrasion, blister, or shallow crater

Stage 3:
- Full-thickness skin loss involving damage to or necrosis of subcutaneous tissue
- May extend down to, but not through, underlying fascia
- Ulcer presents as a deep crater with or without undermining of adjacent tissue

Stage 4:
- Full-thickness skin loss with extensive destruction, tissue necrosis, or damage to muscle, bone, or supporting structures
- May be associated with undermining (spreading underneath) of surrounding tissue and sinus tracts

How it is caused?

There are many factors that, when combined, act to promote the development of pressure sores/ulcers, including:

- External pressure through direct impression, friction, or shearing forces
- Mattress quality and positioning, as well as moisture that occurs with incontinence or diaphoresis
- Poor nutritional status associated with pressure sores and chronic wounds, especially if the person is dehydrated and/or has a low protein intake that results in less resilient skin and a decrease in the cushioning effects of subcutaneous fat layers
- Immobility associated with advanced Parkinson's, cerebrovascular, or Alzheimer's disease and conditions of the muscular-skeletal system such as severe arthritis
- Advanced age and acute illness that may leave the person immobilized, especially if there are many tubes attached to the person for purposes of fluid provision or respiratory assistance

Suggested approaches and interventions

If the problem is:

- Pressure sore/ulcer
  - Wound assessment on regular basis
    - Consider use of the PUSH tool (National Pressure Ulcer Advisor Panel, 1997)
    - Size and shape
    - Wound edges
    - Surrounding skin
    - Ulcer bed
      - Tissue colour
      - Exudates
  - Appropriate wound treatment
    - Cleansing and irrigation, using normal saline or special wound cleansers
    - Avoid topical agents that may impair wound healing
      - If wound healing is not a realistic goal, these agents may be considered to control bacterial load
    - Mechanical, autolytic, or chemical debridement when appropriate
      - Aggressive debridement is not appropriate if complete healing of the wound is not a realistic goal
    - Apply appropriate wound dressing (see wound dressing)
      - Provide adequate pain control if dressing changes cause discomfort

- Fungating wounds
  - Develop in the following cancers:
    - Breast
    - Head and neck
    - Skin
    - Vulva
  - Control tumour growth if possible
    - Chemotherapy
    - Radiation
    - Surgery
  - Control odour
    - Use odour-absorbent dressings
    - Use air-freshening unit and pleasant aromas
    - Place activated charcoal or kitty litter under individual's bed
    - Consider use of aromatherapy
    - If anaerobic infection is causing odour
      - Topical metronidazole
        - Can use metronidazole IV solution mixed with 50 ml normal saline and spray onto lesions
        - Prevents buildup that can occur with metronidazole gel or cream
      - If topical metronidazole fails, consider oral metronidazole
  - Control bleeding
    - Topical thromboplastin 1,000–5,000 units sprayed on area
    - Use padding and haemostatic dressings
    - Consider use of silver sulphadiazine or sucralfate paste
    - Give cyclokapron either crushed into normal saline to make a paste and apply on the wound or as tablet, 500 mg po or as a retention enema; 1000 mg pr
    - If risk of tumour invading vessel, prepare caregivers. Have a written plan in place should major bleeding occur, and escort the family from the room.
      - Provide analgesic and sedative medication q 10 min via IV
        - Administer the prescribed breakthrough analgesic via sc route (if no IV access), repeat q 10 minutes if necessary
        - If opioid naive, administer morphine 5 mg sc and repeat q 20 minutes, if necessary
        - Midazolam 5 mg sc, may repeat q 10 minutes if necessary to control agitation
    - Use dark-coloured blankets or towels to cover individual

- Caregivers and family will require support following event
  - See above re: cyclokapron

- Wound dressings
  - Semipermeable adhesive films (transparent films)
    - Primary dressing:
      - Shallow wound with no exudates
      - Protectant
    - Secondary dressing:
      - Cover other dressing
  - Hydrocolloids
    - Wounds with mild to moderate exudates; not appropriate if heavy exudate
    - Contraindicated if wound infected with anaerobic organisms
    - Promotes autolytic debridement
  - Absorptive dressing
    - Alginates
      - Wounds with mild to heavy exudates
      - Bleeding wounds
    - Foams
      - Wounds with moderate to heavy exudates
      - Allergies to some foam products reported
    - Hydrofibres
      - Wounds with moderate to heavy exudate
  - Odour-absorbent
    - Malodorous wounds
    - Fungating wounds
    - Odorous, exudating bleeding wounds

It is important to keep in mind that wound procedures and repositioning can cause significant pain. Pain assessment should be conducted prior to and during wound procedures such as dressing changes and debridement. In persons suffering from late-stage dementia who may not be able to express their degree of pain, special assessment scales have been developed to try to assess the degree of pain so that nonverbal cues can be used. This often is also suitable for those who are aphasic but might be able to indicate through charts and pictures their degree of pain and discomfort. Chronic pain secondary to wounds should also be evaluated. When a person experiences pain secondary to wound procedures or from pressure sores, they should be provided with appropriate analgesia using various accepted protocols including the World Health Organization (WHO) stepladder.

Appropriate goals for wound healing should be determined, since complete wound healing may not be realistic. If this is the case, it is important to set other appropriate goals, such as providing adequate pain control for wound-related discomfort and preventing systemic complications (such as septicemia) or progression of the wound.

In order to prevent chronic wounds such as pressure sores, it is important to identify at-risk individuals by performing a systematic risk assessment using validated assessment tools such as the Norton (1975) or Braden (1994) scales. Risk should be reassessed at regular intervals.

While reducing pressure is important, this risk must be balanced with patient comfort during repositioning. Provide analgesics if the person experiences pain during this process. Short-acting narcotics should be used in this case, such as SL Fentanyl (25–50mcg of IV Fentanyl preparation) held under tongue for 2 minutes. Wait 5–10 minutes, then reposition the patient.

If the individual is bed bound, repositioning every 2–3 hours is suggested. Pillows or foam wedges can be used to keep bony prominences from direct contact. Devices can also be used to relieve pressure on heels. While in the side-lying position, avoid positioning directly on the trochanter. It can be helpful to reduce amount of time the head of the bed is elevated, as much as the individual's medical condition will allow, to reduce shearing forces. Use lifting devices rather than dragging individuals during transfers and position changes to reduce friction and shearing damage to the skin. Pressure-reducing mattresses, of which there are many, can be helpful. All donut-type devices should be avoided.

If the individual is chair bound, repositioning every 1–2 hours is suggested. The person should be encouraged to shift their weight every 15 minutes between repositioning. This may not be easy to arrange in those with late-stage dementia, as lack of awareness may be a problem. Use pressure-reducing devices for seating surfaces and avoid donut-type devices. The appropriate professional (occupational therapist, physiotherapist) should be consulted regarding posture alignment, weight distribution, balance and stability, and pressure relief when positioning individuals. Specially designed wheelchairs are sometimes helpful if it is recognized that the person will be seated in one for long periods of time to maximize mobility for the person. This also relieves caregivers of frequently moving the person from bed to the sitting position in a chair. For individuals remaining in bed or those who are able to sit in a chair, a written plan should be available to which all caregivers can refer.

Skin care is another area of importance. The skin should be carefully inspected at least once a day while providing care and a bathing schedule should be developed. When bathing, use tepid, not hot, water and a mild, non-abrasive skin cleanser or soap. While many people find massage helpful for muscle pain, do not massage over bony prominences. Environmental factors that contribute to skin breakdown should be minimized, such as low humidity and exposure to cold air. Moisturizers can be used for dry skin, and skin should be cleaned at the time of soiling if the person is incontinent. If incontinence is present, use a moisture barrier following cleansing and use under-pads or briefs that are adsorbent and present a quick-drying surface to the skin.

Dehydration

What does it look like?

Individuals may be suspected of being dehydrated if there is:
- decreased or no urine output
- confusion
- dizziness
- weakness or fatigue
- poor skin turgor
- complaints of thirst or dry mouth

In individuals with late-stage dementia and underlying confusion, it may be difficult to see incremental and subtle changes indicating dehydration. Special attention must be paid to risk factors that may promote dehydration, such as very hot weather with high humidity, especially in situations where there is inadequate climate control.

It is important to keep in mind that dehydration may occur even in the presence of what appears to be excess fluid accumulation in certain parts of the body, such as ascites or peripheral or pulmonary edema.

How it is caused?

Common causes of dehydration include:
- reduced fluid intake
- vomiting
- use of diuretics
- diarrhea
- febrile illnesses with loss of fluids due to perspiration
- very hot weather in the absence of adequate climate control

Suggested approaches and interventions

Please note that the issue of dehydration and the need for rehydration requires thoughtful discussion with the person and their family, as the issue of food and fluid has important personal and cultural meaning to some individuals. In keeping with the palliative care approach, consider subcutaneous hydration very carefully; weigh the benefits and human and emotional repercussions. When possible, speak with individuals about these kinds of controversial issues when they still have the ability to help direct their own destiny rather than trying to predict what they would have wanted when they no longer possess the vital ability to communicate.

If the problem is:

- Dehydration
    - Offer salt (sodium)-containing oral fluids if tolerated
        - Club soda
        - Tomato-based juices
        - Commercial salt and fluid replacement beverages
        - Avoid alcohol and caffeine-containing beverages (e.g., coffee, tea, colas), as these an act as diuretics and increase fluid loss
    - Fluids with minimal salt content
        - Water (must be careful to not over-hydrate, especially in very hot weather conditions, thereby causing low-sodium states (hyponatremia), which can increase the state of confusion in those already suffering from the cognitive effects of late-stage dementia
        - Flat ginger ale
        - Juices (not tomato-based)
    - If subcutaneous hydration (hypodermoclysis) is recommended and agreed to by the afflicted individual and/or his/her family (see note above), use:
        - Normal saline (or 2/3–1/3)
        - Begin infusion at 50 ml/hr and titrate rate according to local tolerance at site and fluid requirements
        - Do not add medications
            - An exception is potassium chloride up to 10 mmol/L
        - Preferred placement sites
            - Scapular or pectoral areas
            - Anterior or lateral aspect of thigh
            - Lateral abdominal wall

- Avoid suprapubic area or 2-inch area around umbilicus
  - Rotate infusion site every 72–96 hours
- Dry Mucous Membranes
  - Eyes
    - Keep conjunctiva moist with:
      - Ocular lubricant q4h
      - Artificial tears 2 drops to each eye q1h pm, especially if eyes are open
  - Lips and nostrils
    - Reduce evaporation by applying thin layer of petroleum jelly
    - Avoid petroleum jelly with plastic tubing (i.e., nasal prongs), as it breaks down the plastic. Use water-based gel.
  - Mouth
    - Chew sugarless gum
    - Suck on hard, sugarless lozenges or sour candies
    - Biotene gel
    - Suck on ice chips or popsicles
    - Frequent sips of water
    - Cool mist vaporizer to increase environmental humidity
      - Clean vaporizer daily
    - Avoid acidic foods/fluids (e.g., orange juice)
    - Regular mouth care to keep mucous membranes and teeth moist and clean
    - Use baking soda mouthwash
      - 1 tsp baking soda, 1 tsp salt, 1 quart tepid water
    - Avoid alcohol-containing mouthwashes, which have a drying effect and may be irritating
    - Commercial artificial saliva substitutes (sprays, swabs, or gel) applied to lips and inner mouth q 1h prn
    - Avoid lemon-glycerin swabs for mouth care, as glycerin is drying and lemon can be irritating

Pain

Note that the section following this portion of the book focuses heavily on issues related to pain management in a setting of palliative care. Although many of the issues are related to palliative care in those with malignant disease, a large number of individuals may also suffer from the effects of cognitive impairment or dementia. There is therefore a considerable overlap in approaches to end-of-life and palliative care in such individuals.
What does it look like?

Pain is an unpleasant sensory or emotional experience derived from sensory stimuli and modified by individual memory, expectations, and emotions.

It is extremely important that you get any information about pain that you can from a patient. Some individuals are reluctant to report their feelings, and untreated pain can result in depression, decreased socialization/ withdrawal, impaired ambulation/decreased mobility, impaired functional ability, and sleep disturbances. In those with late-stage dementia, pain may not be expressed as discomfort but rather as agitation and restlessness. If this is not recognized, the wrong class of medications and interventions may occur. Rather than analgesics being provided, individuals are given various tranquilizing medications, which may decrease their ability to express their discomfort. This can occur without alleviating the pain, which should be avoided whenever possible, as it increases the experience of suffering.

Pain may be described by individuals as:
- Aching
- Burning
- Discomfort
- Heaviness
- "Pins and needles"
- Sharp
- Stabbing
- Stinging
- Tingling
- Tightness

Individuals who have become cognitively impaired, especially in the later stages of dementia, or who have communication difficulties may present with:
- Agitated behavior/restlessness
- Changes in facial expression. A very good indicator of pain and distress across all cultures is furrowing of the brow and/or tension across forehead, as well as clenching of teeth.
- Changes in functional ability
- Changes in gait/decreased mobility
- Verbalizations such as crying, groaning, and moaning

How it is caused?

- **Nociceptive** pain results from stimulation of chemical, pressure, stretch, and temperature receptors (nociceptors) found throughout the body
  - Somatic
    - Usually well-localized
    - Can be constant or intermittent
    - Often described as "gnawing" or "aching"
  - Visceral
    - Usually poorly localized
    - Usually constant
    - Often described as "aching," "squeezing," "penetrating"
- **Neuropathic** pain results from damage or irritation to a specific nerve of group of nerves
  - Dysesthetic is often described as constant burning or "pins and needles"
  - Neuralgic is often described as "sharp," "stabbing," or "shooting" pain with an "electrical feel"

Common causes of nociceptive pain in older individuals include:
- Arthropathies (pain from joint disease)
- Malignancy
- Myalgias (pain from muscles)
- Skin and mucosal ulcerations
- Non-articular inflammatory disorders from parts of the body other than joints
- Cardiovascular disease

Neuropathic pain may be caused by the following conditions:
- Post-herpetic pain (after an attack of *herpes zoster*—shingles)
- Diabetic neuropathy
- Post-stroke pain
- Post-amputation pain
- Post-radiation pain
- Post-surgical pain
- Trigeminal neuralgia
- Malignancy
- Nerve impingement

Pain assessment
(For individuals with cognitive impairment or communication difficulties, see page 120 for a visual analogue scale, numerical scale, or descriptive scale.)

Suggested approaches and interventions

Stepwise analgesia as outlined by the World Health Organization

Step 3, Severe Pain (7-10)

Hydromorphone
Methadone
Fentanyl
Oxycodone
± *Nonopioid analgesics*
±*Adjuvants*

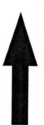

Step 2, Moderate Pain (5-6)

Hydrocodone
Oxycodone
Tramadol
± *Nonopioid analgesics*
±*Adjuvants*

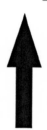

Step 1, Mild Pain (1-4)

Acetaminophen (Acet)
±*Adjuvants*

"Adjuvants" refers either to medications that are coadministered to manage an adverse effect of an opioid, or to so-called adjuvant analgesics that are added to enhance analgesia such as steroids for pain from bone metastases. Adjuvants also includes medication such as anticonvulsants for neuropathic pain.

Note that codeine has been added by new consensus guidelines for non-malignant pain, along with tramadol (Ultram).

If the problem is:
- Arthritic pain
    - Consult physiotherapy if that is possible and available
        - Provide a specific exercise plan to strengthen muscles and minimize gait disorders if the person is able to cooperate at that level
        - Assess mobility and evaluate need for mobility aids if the person is still able to be mobile and ambulate
        - Evaluate TENS, which is not always possible in those suffering from late-stage dementia
        - Assess for appropriateness of thermal therapy, which may not be available to many people with late-stage dementia
    - Medications
        - Step one
            - Acetaminophen 325–650 mg po q 4–6h on a round-the-clock basis
                - Maximum dose generally set at 3000 mg per 24 hours (although sometimes a dose 4000 mg/24 hours is used for defined period)
            - NSAIDs
                - Issue in renal disease
                - Considered second- or third-line agents due to potential adverse effects
                - Some clinicians would recommend the addition of codeine or tramadol before considering NSAIDs.
                - NSAIDs may be more effective than acetaminophen, codeine or tramadol if clear cut inflammation is present
                - Add cytoprotective agent if high risk for NSAID-related GI ulceration
                - Misoprostol (Cytotec) 200 ug pot id-qid (not usually added as single agent; Arthrotec has the misoprostol with diclofenac)
                - Proton pump inhibitor
                - Ranitidine
            - COX-2 specific NSAIDs (probably preferable in all situations to the use of a usual NSAID)
                - May be lower risk of NSAID-related GI ulceration, although long-term data in frail seniors, especially those with late-stage dementia, are not available. Other adverse affects such as

fluid retention and elevated blood pressure occur
with all of the NSAIDs.
- Step two
  - Add codeine to above
    - Codeine 15–30 mg prn, or use a combination with
      the acetaminophen (i.e., #1, 2, 3; each contain a
      fixed dose of codeine with the acetaminophen)
      until the effective does is determined, and then
      switch to regular dosing
    - Remember to include a stimulant or osmotic
      laxative regimen to prevent opioid-related
      constipation
- Step three
  - If inadequate response, discontinue codeine and
    rotate to tramadol (according to recently updated
    guidelines)
  - If inadequate, add stronger opioid
  - Morphine 2.5–5 mg po q 4h
  - Hydromorphine 1 mg po q 4h
  - Oxycodone 2.5–5 mg po q 4h (oxycodone is twice
    as potent as morphine, so start with 2.5 mg only)
  - Long-acting opioids may be used to simplify the
    dosing regimen when satisfactory pain control is
    achieved

- Neuropathic pain
  - Consult physiotherapy if possible and available
    - Evaluation of TENS if the person is able to cooperate and
      participate
    - Determine appropriate exercise program to minimize
      myofascial complications associated with neuropathic pain
  - Based on degree of severity, optimize other analgesics during
    titration period and decrease dose of these agents as pain control
    allows
  - Determine dysesthetic-type pain, if possible, from adequate history
    or previous information (i.e., long history prior to the progress of
    the dementia)
    - Tricyclic antidepressants
      - Desipramine or nortriptyline have lower anticholinergic
        effects than amitriptyline

- Initiate at 10–25 mg po qhs and titrate dose every 5–7 days by 10–25 mg as tolerated
- 75–100 mg usual maximum daily dose for pain
  - Gabapentin (Neuorontin)
    - 100 mg po tid (start even lower in elderly eg 100 mg qhs, then 100 q 12h then q 8h
    - Titrate by 100 mg tid every 3–5 days as tolerated
    - 600 mg tid usual maximum daily dose for seniors
    - Works well in combination with tricyclic antidepressants
    - Dose dependant on renal function
  - Pregabalin (Lyrica)
    - 50 mg po bid to start
    - Titrate by 50 mg every 3–5 days as tolerated
    - 450 mg/day is maximum dose (may not be tolerated at high doses in people with dementia)
    - Dose dependant on renal function
  - SNRIs (duloxetine; start at 30 mg od, max dose 60 mg/day)
  - Methadone; depending on the jurisdiction, you may need special license
  - Sativex spray
  - Capsaicin
    - 0.025–0.075% cream applied to affected areas tid-qid
    - Burning associated with application when initiated is transient and decreases with in 14 days
    - Wash hands immediately following application
    - Avoid contact with eyes
    - Not recommended if delirium or severe cognitive impairment
- Consider referral for nerve block
- Consider radiotherapy if related to malignancy (i.e., nerve compression)
- Consider referral to palliative care specialist if pain persists
- Bone pain
  - Provide stepwise analgesia according to severity rating
    - NSAIDs can be helpful, but side effects may limit their use
    - The role of COX-2 specific agents has not been defined for bone pain related to malignancy
  - Consider addition of dexamethasone 2–4 mg po if bone metastases or there is nerve impingement
  - Depending on prognosis, consider adding a bisphosphonate if breast cancer or malignant myeloma with bone metastases

- Consider referral for radiotherapy if localized bone pain is secondary to bone metastases
- Calcitonin 100–200 IU sc or intranasally if pain related to vertebral fracture
  - Can administer test dose 25 IU sc to determine if allergic
- Refer to palliative care specialist if pain persists

Medication and dosage forms (please refer to charts in next section of guide).

Consider use of other treatment modalities when appropriate, including palliative radiotherapy and chemotherapy. Caregivers should also think about using non-pharmacologic modalities, like physiotherapy, music therapy, art therapy, relaxation therapy, and therapeutic touch. In any case, treatment should address all aspects of suffering: physical, psychosocial, cultural, and spiritual. Caregivers should, of course, monitor the effectiveness of treatment plan on a regular basis.

For medications, consider the following: The oral route is the preferred route of administration, unless individual is experiencing severe nausea/vomiting or is unable to swallow. Try to avoid intramuscular injections, as they can be painful and use subcutaneous route for parenteral administration. Use "round-the-clock" dosing for individuals who describe or indicate constant pain. Use prn dosing for individuals who describe or indicate intermittent pain or for breakthrough pain for people receiving "round-the-clock" medication. Titrate the dose of medication individually: be cautious if person seems to require rapid titration of opioids as they may be expressing total suffering as pain. Determine if other factors are influencing the pain experience. Remember to use adjuvant medications when appropriate

Provide an ongoing education regarding analgesic medications to people with pain, their families, and caregivers. In those suffering from dementia, the focus of education must be the family or others involved in the decision-making process. It is important for them to appreciate the importance of addressing analgesic needs, as pain experienced by those suffering from dementia adds unnecessarily to an already difficult situation. Misconceptions about addiction and tolerance can lead to poor adherence and inadequate pain relief.

Assess symptoms in a systematic and multidimensional fashion. Special skills and talents are required from the caregivers in assessing those suffering from late-stage dementia because of difficulties in clearly expressing the nature and degree of discomfort and pain.

Recognize that individuals in end-stage dementia may describe symptoms in a non-specific manner or sometimes not at all. Finding alternate ways of communicating with them other than verbally is key to the palliative approach to end-stage dementia care. Remember, one of the main goals is to give the individual what he or she wants—that is, to make his or her situation the most comfortable as possible. In order to achieve this, good communication is mandatory.

Medications have side effects, so it is always important to consider the risks and benefits of pain medications in these circumstances. Always weigh the benefits and costs of administering the specific drug in your specific situation, and try non-pharmacological interventions where you can.

Appendix B:
Useful Scales, Assesment Tools, and Medications for Symptom Management

Although many of these scales have been developed for those experiencing malignant and non-malignant pain rather than those living with dementia, there is often an overlap between those with dementia and those with serious pain. It is a special challenge to assess individuals living with dementia, especially during the late stages of their disease, to determine their painful symptoms and what combination of interventions might be suitable for them. Other symptoms, such as agitation, whether from pain or other reasons, can also present a considerable therapeutic challenge. The recommendations in this section should be seen as a guide to help clinicians in their decision-making, with the final decisions of therapeutic intervention being tailored by the clinician to the specific situation of the patient in question.

It is also important to remember that, depending on the stage of dementia and where the person is in on the trajectory of decline, different approaches might be more suitable for one situation than another. Those individuals who are already bed bound and completely dependant, with a severely compromised level of function, might benefit from levels of pain control that might not be suitable for someone who is still mobile and would like to remain so for as long as possible and who is able to tolerate pain to a greater degree than the bed-bound person.

Pain Assessment Scales

There are many pain assessment scales in use. The ones demonstrated below are examples of those commonly used in the palliative care community and might be useful in some individuals who suffer from cognitive impairment or dementia.

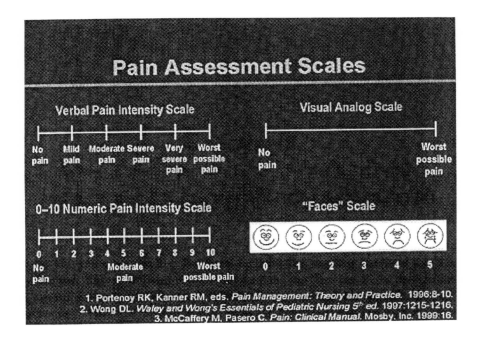

Pain Assessment Scales

Verbal Pain Intensity Scale

No pain · Mild pain · Moderate pain · Severe pain · Very severe pain · Worst possible pain

Visual Analog Scale

No pain — Worst possible pain

0–10 Numeric Pain Intensity Scale

0 1 2 3 4 5 6 7 8 9 10
No pain · Moderate pain · Worst possible pain

"Faces" Scale

0 1 2 3 4 5

1. Portenoy RK, Kanner RM, eds. *Pain Management: Theory and Practice.* 1996:8-10.
2. Wong DL. *Waley and Wong's Essentials of Pediatric Nursing 5ᵗʰ ed.* 1997:1215-1216.
3. McCaffery M, Pasero C. *Pain: Clinical Manual.* Mosby. Inc. 1999:16.

Approach to the introduction of pain management, depending on level of pain and response to intervention (Some of the points in this section have been made in the previous section, but this duplication was intended to avoid the necessity of going back and forth between sections of the guide.)

Analgesics: Non-Opioids: NSAIDs, acetaminophen
Weak Opioids: codeine, Tramadol (an atypical opioid)
Strong Opioids: morphine, oxycodone, hydromorphone and fentanyl (**never use fentanyl patch in opioid naïve patients**)

Pharmacologic Adjuvant (used to promote the effectiveness of another drug when used in combination with it): antidepressants, anticonvulsants, corticosterioids, bisphosphonates, local anesthetics, antispasmodics, palliative chemotherapy, NSAIDs.

Non-pharmacologic Adjuvant: radiation therapy, acupuncture, TENS, ultrasound, therapeutic touch, massage, splints, surgery, counseling, cognitive behavior therapy, music and art therapy, relaxation techniques.

Symptom Management

This section includes the updated version of the Baycrest publication *Palliative Care Handbook*, 2011, Baycrest Geriatric Health Care System, Toronto, authored by Grossman D, Kirstein A, Buchman D, Buchman S, Gordon M (2011).

Opioid Dosing Table

Group	Drug	Strengths Available	Suggested Dosing Interval	Onset of Action (minutes)
Codeine	Codeine Tablets	15 mg, 30 mg	Q 4h	15–30
	Codeine Syrup	5 mg/ml	Q 4h	15–30
	Codeine Contin (long acting)	50 mg, 100 mg	Q 8–12h	Peaks in 1–2 hours
	Codeine Injection	30 mg/ml	Q 4h	10–30
Tramadol	Ultram and Ultram ER	Ultram 50 mg and Ultram ER: 100, 200, 300 mg	Ultram 50–100 mg q 4–6 h Ultram ER 100–300 mg/day	30–60
Morphine	Morphine tabs	5, 10, 25, 50 mg	Q 4h	10–30
	Morphine syrup	1 mg/ml	Q 4h	10–30
	M-Eslon (long-acting Morphine)	10, 15, 30, 60, 100 (mg)	Q 8–12h	Peaks in 3–4 hours
	Morphine Injection	2 mg/ml, 10 mg/ml, 15 mg/ml, 50 mg/ml, 250 mg/5ml, 500 mg/10ml	Q 4h or CSCI	15–60
Hydromorphone	Hydromorphone Tabs *(Dilaudid)*	1, 2, 4, 8 (mg)	Q 4h	15–30
	Hydromorphone Contin (long acting)	3, 12, 24, 30 (mg)	Q8-12h	Peaks at mean of 4–8 hours
	Hydromorphone Injection *(Dilaudid)*	2mg/ml, 10mg/ml, 50mg/5ml, 100mg/50ml, 500mg/50ml, 2500mg/50ml	Q4h or CSCI	10–15

Oxycodone	Oxycodone	5, 10 mg	Q4h	10–15
	Oxycocet	Acetaminophen 325 mg/ oxycodone 5 mg	Q 4h	10–15
	OxyContin (long acting Oxycodone)	10, 20, 80 mg	Q 8–12h	Peaks in 2.8 hours
Fentanyl	Fentanyl Patch	12, 25, 50, 75, 100 (µg)	Q 3–days	Following administration, serum concentration levels off between 12–24 hours. Steady state reached in approx. 2–3 days

DO NOT USE fentanyl patch in opioid-naïve patients

Equianalgesic Chart

P.O : S.C : IV = 1 : 2 : 3

Drug	P.O. mg	S.C. mg	IV mg	Schedule
Morphine	20	10	6	Q 4h
Hydromorphone	4	2	1–2	Q 4h
Oxycodone	10	N/A	N/A	Q 4h
Codeine	200	100	50–100	Q 4h
Fentanyl Patch	*25 µg/hr fentanyl ≈ 60 mg oral morphine/24 hours			Q 3 days

- *Health Canada says that the equivalent is 120 mg morphine, but palliative care physician community does not agree and prefers the lower dose equivalent.
- 10% of population cannot convert codeine to morphine; for these people, codeine is not effective at all.

Rules of Thumb
- When converting from one opioid to another, decrease the equivalency dose by 30–50% because of incomplete cross-tolerance.

Example: codeine 80 mg po q 4h
Codeine to morphine = 10:1
Therefore: codeine 80 mg po q 4h = morphine 8 mg po q 4h

To account for incomplete cross-tolerance, reduce this dose by 30%, making the starting dose morphine 5 mg po q 4h.

Longer-Acting Opioids

- Sustained release (SR) preparations should not be used for uncontrolled pain or in patients whose opioid needs have not yet been determined. Always titrate with short-acting and convert to long-acting when the appropriate dose is reached.

- Slow-release preparations of morphine (MS Contin, M-Eslon, MOS-SR, Oramorph SR), hydromorphone (Hydropmorph Contin), codeine (Codeine Contin), and oxycodone (OxyContin): calculate total 24-hour dose (oral equivalent), divide by 2, and administer q 12 hr regularly. If pain repeatedly recurs before 12 hours, increase dose or shorten interval to q 8h.

- **Transdermal fentanyl** *(Duragesic)*: continuous release for 72 hours. Calculate oral morphine (mg/day) equivalency and apply appropriate dose of patch (µg/hr).

Example: If the patient is controlled on morphine 5 mg po q 4h, then the total 24-hour dose of morphine = 30 mg. The patient can be converted to M-Eslon 15 mg po bid.

Breakthrough Pain Medication

It is extremely important when titrating the dosage of an opioid analgesic to supply the patient with sufficient "breakthrough" pain medication, also referred to as "rescue" medication. The dosage of rescue medication is generally 10–20% of the total daily dose of opioid at an interval of q 1h prn.

- The breakthrough dose is approximately 10% of the total 24-hour dose. Regular use of 2 or more prn (breakthrough) doses in 24 hours indicates inadequate pain control. The background opioid dose needs to be adjusted accordingly.

Example: If the patient is taking morphine 5 mg po q 4h (30 mg per day), then the breakthrough dose would be 2.5 mg po q 1h prn. If the patient is converted to M-Eslon 15 mg po bid, the hourly breakthrough dose would still be 2.5 mg po q 1h prn.

If the patient is no longer able to take oral medication: Indication for sc/iv use.

PO: SC dose = 2: 1
Therefore Morphine 5 mg po q 4h = Morphine 2.5 mg sc q 4h
Breakthrough: Morphine 2.5 mg po q 1h prn = Morphine 1 mg sc q 1h prn

Bone Pain

Bone pain is often due to metastatic malignant disease with tumours in the bones, and is felt as a localized aching.

Medications:
- Opioid
- ± NSAID or COX_2
- Steroid (if unable to tolerate NSAID or prior to radiotherapy)

Bisphosphanates:
- Clodronate *(Bonefos)*—800 mg bid po
- Pamidronate *(Aredia)*—90 mg IV infused over 3 hours once/month
- Zolendranate IV if the pain is refractory to the above

For metastatic breast cancer and multiple myeloma, consider:
- Radiotherapy
- Splinting
- Surgical fixation (under unusual circumstances)

Medications used in adjuvant therapy:
- Tricyclic antidepressants
- Nortriptyline, amitriptyline (cyclic drugs)

Nortriptyline has fewer anticholenergic side effects than amitriptyline, and it can significantly reduce blood pressure.
Start at 10 to 25 mg po qhs. Increase dose q 3–5 days by 10–25 mg as tolerated (max 75–150 mg od).

Anticonvulsants for Neuropathic Pain

Drugs	Dosage	Adverse Effects	Comments
Gabapentin *(Neurontin)*	• 100–300 mg po on day 1: (once/day) • Day 2: (bid) • Day 3 (tid)	Sedation	Max = 3600 mg/day (often use less in those suffering from late-stage dementia)
Pregabalin *(Lyrica)*	• 25–50 mg up to tid	Sedation	Max = 300 mg/day (often use less in those suffering from late-stage dementia)
Valproic acid *(Depakene, Epival)*	250 to 500 mg hs increasing to 1000 to 1500 mg hs; can be given pr	Sedation, thrombocytopenia	
Carbamazepine *(Tegretol)*	100 to 200 mg bid increasing slowly to a maximum of 400 mg tid	Drowsiness, nausea, interaction with anti-depressants may increase effects of both	May monitor blood levels
Clonazepam *(Rivotril)*	0.5 mg hs increasing to 2 to 3 mg max daily	Drowsiness common and limiting	May be useful

In elderly patients, especially those with dementia, the starting doses are adjusted to lower levels.

Other supplementary treatments:
• SNRIs—Duloxetine
• Cannabinoids (Sativex buccal spray)
• methadone
• Nerve block
• Epidural
• Transcutaneous Electronic Nerve Stimulation (TENS)

Anti-inflammatory medications often used along with analgesics include dexamethasone *(Decadron)* 4 mg po/sc qid.

Controlling Opioid Side Effects

It is important to anticipate opioid side effects: these include drowsiness, which may be transient and usually resolves after 2-3 days. Remember the relationship between various routes of administration is PO/IV/SC; dose is 2:1:06. When rotating opioids, decrease the equivalency dose by 30–50% because of incomplete cross tolerance. Avoid Morphine in renal failure. Hydromorphone is a better choice. **Never use IM route.** Nausea and vomiting occur in 50 to 70% of patients exposed to opioids; therefore order an anti-emetic along with the opioid, unless the previous exposure to strong opioids has not produced nausea in the patient. Remember that many patients require prn doses of anti-emetics. Those with chronic nausea will require round-the-clock dosing.

Suggested Anti-emetics for Opioid-induced Nausea

Drug	Dosage	Comments
First-Line Agent		
Metoclopramide (*Maxeran*)	5–10 mg po or sc q 1h prn up to 80 mg/day 5–20 mg po tid ½ hr ac + qhs	Adverse effects can include extra-pyramidal symptoms
Haloperidol (*Haldol*)	0.5–2 mg sc or po up to q 1h prn. Not to exceed 16 mg/d	Adverse effects rare at low dose; can cause extra-pyramidal symptoms
Secondary Drug		
Prochlorperazine (*Stemetil*)	5–10 mg pr or po q 4h prn	Dystonic effects and sedation may occur
Other Drugs		
Chlorpromazine (*Largactil*)	25–50 mg po q 6h prn	Dystonic effects and sedation may occur
Methotrimeprazine (*Nozinan*)	2.5mg–25mg q2-4h prn po/sc	Dystonic effects and sedation may occur
Dimenhydrinate (*Gravol*)	25–50 mg pr or po q 4–6h prn	Especially if vertigo present; sedation may occur

If stomach motility seems to be an issue, or if a first-line drug is ineffective, try adding motility agents.

Motility Agents

Drug	Dosage	Comments
Metoclopramide (*Maxeran*)	5–20 mg qid ½ hour AC + qhs	Adverse effects can include extra-pyramidal symptoms; better for nausea
Domperidone (*Motilium*)	10–40 mg qid ½ hour AC + qhs	Give before meals. Not available sc

Constipation

Always anticipate when using opioids. You should optimize diet, fluids, exercise, and privacy. Reassess daily and adjust laxatives as necessary.

Medications to treat:

Senna (*Senokot*)	2–4 tabs od bid Max 8 tablets/day
Bisacodyl (*Dulcolax*)	5 mg po, 10 mg pr once/daily
Lactulose (*Chronulac, Cephlac*)	30–60 cc od tid
Propylene Glycol	Lax-a-day, MiraLAX and RestoraLAX : 17 gm/day prn and for no more than 7 days in a row
Docusate (*Colace*)	100–200 bid (do not use as single agent)
Glycerine Suppository	1 prn
Enemas (*Fleet Enema*)	prn

Where maximum doses of laxatives have failed and the patient is not taking anything by mouth, and where rectal administration of enemas and suppositories are not possible, Methylnaltrexone (Relistor—dosing is by patient's weight) given subcutaneously may be indicated. It is contraindicated in complete bowel obstruction, but may be considered in partial obstruction, as per physician judgment and discretion.

Myoclonic Jerks

Myoclonic jerks are brief, involuntary muscle jerks that can be painful. Consider a reversible cause where possible, e.g. dehydration, electrolyte imbalances (Na, K, Ca, Mg), infection, or medications, e.g. opioids (especially when dose increased rapidly). Also consider new medications altering the metabolism of opioids.

If the problem is opioid related, attempt to the reduce dose, rehydrate patient if possible, and then attempt to rotate the opioid.

Medications to treat:

Lorazepam *(Ativan)*	0.5–1 mg sc/po/sl q 4h prn
Diazepam *(Valium)*	2.5–5 mg po q 8–12 hours
Clonazepam *(Rivotril)*	0.25–0.5 mg po bid – tid
Midazolam *(Versed)*	0.5 mg sc q 20 min prn

Respiratory Depression

Protocol for the Administration of SC Naloxone (Narcan) for the Management of Opioid-Induced Respiratory Depression in Patients Receiving Opioids via PCA

Goal: To reverse respiratory depression without reversal of analgesia.

To avoid pain-crisis and withdrawal-reaction:

If respiratory rate is >10 per minute and sedation score = 3, then hold opioid

If respiratory rate <10 per minute and sedation score >=, 3 then see next section: emergency reversal of opiod-induced respiratory depression

Sedation Scale

```
0 = none; alert patient
1 = mild; occasionally drowsy patient, but easy to arouse
2 = moderate; increased drowsiness, but still easy to arouse
3 = severe; somnolent patient, difficult to arouse
S = sleep; patient is asleep and is easily aroused with stimulation
```

Purpose: Emergency reversal of opioid-induced respiratory depression

Patient Population: Patients who are receiving opioids

Indication: Reversal of respiratory depression characterized by both of the following:

Respiratory rate <10 per minute

AND

Sedation scale of 3 (decreased level of consciousness, difficult to rouse)

Contraindications:
- Patients who are awake
- Patients who are sedated but easy to rouse, regardless of the respiratory rate.

Management Protocol:
1. Stop opioid.
2. Notify physician.
3. Administer O_2 5L/min via nasal prongs.
4. Nurse to monitor the following:
   Respiratory rate
   Blood pressure
   Heart rate
   Level of consciousness (sedation scale)
5. Have equipment ready to start hydration if indicated.
6. Administer naloxone: select ampoule containing naloxone 0.4 mg per 1 ml; dilute to 10 ml with normal saline to give 0.04 mg/ml (9 ml of NS + 0.4 mg/ml Naloxone); give 0.04 mg (1 mL) SC or IV over 5 seconds.
7. Wait 5 minutes. Repeat vital signs. If respiratory rate <10/min and sedation scale >3, give a second dose of Naloxone 0.08 mg (2 ml) sc or iv over 5 seconds.
8. Wait 5 minutes. Repeat vital signs. If respiratory rate <10/min and sedation scale = 3, give another dose of naloxone 0.08 mg (2 ml) sc or iv over 5 seconds.
9. Continue vital signs every 15 minutes until patient condition stable or otherwise specified by physician.

Naloxone has a short half-life. If patient responds to 0.1 mg, they may need either a naloxone drip or a naloxone 0.1 mg sc or iv q 1h PRN until respiratory rate or sedation score stabilizes.

Note: During chronic opioid therapy (e.g., cancer pain), small doses of naloxone are recommended to avoid withdrawal reactions and re-emergence of pain.

Skin Care

Pruritis

Topically:
- Consider non-allergenic sheets
- Mild soaps
- Moisturizer
- Menthol/camphor
- Topical steroids
- Doxepin topical cream

Oral Medications to treat:

Doxepin *(Sinequan)*	Start at 10 mg hs and titrate upward
Cholestyramine *(Questran)*	If jaundiced, 4 gm po tid
Oral antihistamines	Diphenhydramine (Benadryl) 50 mg po q 6h hydroxyzine (Atarax) 25 mg q 8h
Mirtazapine (Remeron)	7.5 mg–15 mg qhs
Dexamethasone (Decadron)	0.5–1.0 mg once or twice daily
Paroxetine	10–20 mg/day

Skin Breakdown

To prevent skin breakdown: turn q 2h, use a pressure relief mattress (Therarest, Advance 2000) and protect normal skin with barrier cream or moisturizer

Stage	Skin Breakdown	Rx
1	Non-blanchable erythema—intact skin The skin will show apparent redness over pressure point(s) that does not fade 30–45 minutes after relief of pressure. This is reversible with intervention.	1. Cleanse with normal saline; apply Tegaderm or Opsite to protect from shearing forces. 2. Apply transparent film dressing or thin hydrocolloid dressing. May use liquid skin sealant to promote better adhesion of dressing.
2	Superficial break in epidermis and dermis. There is no necrotic tissue. Observe for skin loss, edema, colour, location, depth and size. May have linear split, viable flap, or dead skin flap. Fluid filled intact blister.	1. Clean with normal saline and pat dry with dry sterile gauze. 2. Abrasions. Apply hydrocolloid dressing (Duoderm). Change every 2–3 days if dead skin tissue is present or every 4–6 days if wound is clean. 3. Skin Tears and Blisters: Apply non-adherent dressing. Change every 3–4 days.

3	Full thickness skin loss involving damage or necrosis of subcutaneous tissue that may extend down to fascia.	Cleanse area with normal saline. Protect surrounding skin from maceration with plasticized film coating (e.g., Skin Prep).
	Look for thick, black eschar (possibly brown or grey). The wound may be partially or completely covered with eschar, or with "string like" slough, or with loose necrotic tissue, which may be brown or grey in colour.	Use one of these methods to remove the dead tissue: • Surgical Debridement: Use scalpel, scissors, or other sharp instrument to remove dead tissue. This is the most effective and fastest means of removing dead tissue. • Done only by a physician or an Advanced Practice Nurse with additional education either at the bedside, as in cases of small ulcers, or at the clinic. • Generally indicated when there is an urgent need for debridement (e.g., in cases of advancing cellulitis or sepsis).
	Assess for blood supply to ensure healing ability of the wound. (Debridement is contraindicated if there is poor blood supply.)	• Autolytic debridement: Apply hydrogel (e.g., Intrasite Gel) to necrotic area, ensuring that the entire wound is completely covered. If the eschar is thick, crosshatch the eschar to facilitate penetration of gel into the eschar. Cover with semi-occlusive dressing (e.g., hydrocolloid or foam dressing), fastened by dressing retention sheets (e.g., Mefix, Hypafix, Opsite).

| | | • For smaller necrotic areas, or wounds with relatively thin eschar, a small amount of Intrasite Gel covered with Opsite may be effective.
• Change dressing every 24–72 hours to remove liquefied necrotic material. Do not leave the dressing longer than 3 days.

• Enzymatic debridement. Accomplished by application of topical debriding agents to necrotic tissues on the wound surface. Collagenase (Santyl) is an example of this agent.

Attending physician and assess for antibiotics. |
| | Granulating (Red) Wound

Look for bright-red tissue with slightly bumpy appearance. There may be a small to large amount of sero-sanguinous drainage | Granulating (Red) Wound
1. Clean with normal saline. Ensure that the skin around the wound is clean and dry.
2. In cases where there is large amount of drainage, cover with absorbent dressing (e.g., Mepilex Foam Adhesive or Mepilex border dressing). Change dressing every 1–3 days or prn.
3. Apply/swab surrounding skin with plasticized coating (e.g., Skin Prep) to protect from maceration and irritation from the drainage. |

	Exudating (Yellow) Wound Look for moderate or heavy drainage at the wound site	Exudating (Yellow) Wound 1. Clean with normal saline. Ensure that the skin around the wound is clean and dry. 2. If wound is draining a small amount, cover with hydrocolloid dressing (e.g., Mepilex/Tegasorb). 3. If wound is draining a moderate to large amount, cover with absorbent foam dressing (e.g., Mepilex adhesive or Mepilex border). Change dressing as needed according to saturation of exudate on the dressing.
4	Full-thickness skin loss with extensive destruction of tissue, necrosis, or damage to muscle, bone, or supporting structures. Wound presents as a deep crater or cavity. May either be dry or exudating. May include undermining of sinus formation.	1. Irrigate and clean ulcer bed with normal saline. Use 30-cc syringe with 18-g needle to flush ulcer bed with normal saline. A urethral catheter may be attached to the syringe to flush/irrigate the sinus tract. 2. If cavity is sloughy, line the cavity with hydrogel (Intrasite Gel), and then fill loosely with normal saline and Intrasite-saturated gauze or packing strips and cover with Mepilex adhesive or sheets or dry sterile dressing fastened by dressing retention sheets (e.g., Mefix, Flexifix). 3. If draining heavily, cover with absorbent dressings (e.g., Exu-Dry gauze, Mepilex dressing) and change dressing every 1–2 days and prn. 4. Protect surrounding skin with liquid sealant (e.g., Skin Prep). 5. Implement preventive measures.

Medications:
- Topical Metronidazole gel, cream, or tabs directly on wounds
- Dressing soaked in metronidazole injectable solution
- Metronidazole 500 mg po q 12h

Neurological Symptoms

Rule out underlying causes and treat, if appropriate (e.g. hypercalcemia, electrolyte imbalance, dehydration, constipation, cerebral metastases, infection, hypoxia, urinary retention, drugs).

Delirium and Restlessness

Common medication causes include opioids, anticholinergic medications, and sedatives.

If the problem is opioid induced, consider a reduction in dose or rotation to another opioid.

Medications to treat:

Haloperidol (*Haldol*)	1–2 mg po/sc bid – tid up to q 1h prn
Methotremeprazine (*Nozinan*)	5–25mg po/sc q 4h prn
Chlorpromazine (*Largactil*)	12.5–50 mg po/pr/iv q 8–12 hrs (may be more sedating) Should not give sc
Risperidone (*Risperdal*)	0.5 mg po bid—titrate to effect
Olanzapine/Olanzapine Zydis (*Zyprexa*)	2.5 mg po bid—titrate to effect
Quetiapine (*Seroquel*)	25 mg po qhs—titrate to effect
Lorazepam (*Ativan*)	0.5–1 mg po/sl/sc q1 hrs prn
Midazolam (*Versed*)	0.5–1 mg/hr infusion, with increments as required. Start infusion at 0.5 mg/hr. Give 0.5 mg q 30 prn until sedated. If patient requires 2 x 0.5 mg in 1 hour, increase drip by 0.5 mg/hour. There is no ceiling.

If using benzodiazepines, these should be used in combination with antipsychotic medications. Beware of aggravating agitation with benzodiazepine; it may be necessary to add a low dose of an antipsychotic in such situations, especially in the face of late-stage dementia with behavioural symptoms, which often include agitation.

Seizures

In palliative care situations, it is not always feasible to achieve IV access. Therefore, the management of seizures may have to be achieved through the SC route.

Medications to treat:

Ativan 1 mg sl/sc q 5 min >4 mg
Maintenance 1 mg po/sc/sl q 4–6h

Valium 10 mg PR x 1 dose
Maintenance 5 mg po/pr q 6h

Midazolam 1 mg sc q 10 min until relief, followed by midazolam infusion. If patient is unable to swallow, may increase dose to 5 mg.

Phenobarbital 30–60 mg po/pr/sc q 10 min to maximum of 20 mg/kg
If patient is unable to swallow, initiate phenobarbital at dose of 1–3 mg/kg/day in one to two divided doses, or as CSCI.

If patient is able to swallow, start with Dilantin 200 mg/day hs and adjust dose accordingly.

If hypoglycemia is suspected, then perform stat blood sugar and treat with 50 ml of 50% glucose IV.

If brain metastases are suspected, give dexamethasone 10 mg po/sc/iv stat followed by 4 mg qid urgent referral to radiation therapy, if appropriate.

Cord Compression

Sign		Clinical level	
	Cord	*Conus medullaris*	*Cauda equina*
Motor	Paraparesis usually flaccid Pyramidal signs can be present	Same as cord	Never pyramidal signs Often asymmetrical Weakness
Reflex	Absent or hyperactive	Patellar hyperactive Ankle hypoactive	Hypoactive Asymmetrical
Babinski	Usually present	Usually present	Never present
Sensory	Dermatomal level sensory loss (Locates compression within two dermatomes above the sensory level)	Same as cord (level usually at L1)	Asymmetrical findings in the lower extremities and perineum
Sphincter Control	Can be initially preserved	Early involved Sometimes selectively	Can be preserved

Treatment for acute Cord Compression

Dexamethasone 10 mg po/sc/iv stat then 4 mg po/sc/iv qid. Consider urgent radiation referral to radiation oncology if appropriate and if life expectancy sufficient and symptoms sufficient to merit such intervention.

Mouth Care

Avoid commercial mouthwashes, lemon, glycerin swabs or artificial saliva.

Dry Mouth

Consider:
- Biotene gel (first line)
- Sour candies
- Ice chips, popsicles

- Moisten with water or normal saline (spray bottle, syringe, red rubber catheter)
- KY jelly to inside of mouth
- Petroleum jelly for lips
- Humidifier or humidified air/oxygen
- Moisture spray

Oral Candidiasis

This condition is usually due to antibiotics, steroids, etc.

Medications to treat:

Mycostatin *(Nystatin)*	500,000 units swish and swallow qid x 7 days
If Nystatin Fails...	
Ketoconazole *(Nizoral)*	200 mg po od x 5–7 days
Fluconazole *(Diflucan)*	100 mg po od x 5–7 days

Ulceration and Stomatitis: Medications to treat

Normal saline rinses	q 2 hours
Benzydamine HCl *(Tantum)*	Oral rinse—½ or full strength 15 ml qid
Penicillin	If severe—po/iv
Mycostatin *(Nystatin)*	500,000 units swish and swallow qid (prophylactic)
Xylocaine viscous Or xylocaine:nystatin 1:1 solution	2% to paint mouth, 15 ml q 3h (maximum 120 ml/24 hour); do not eat 1 hr after dose
Antacids *(Maalox)*	Swish and swallow
Sucrulfate Suspension	1 g qid
Sulcrafate:Xylocaine viscous 1:1	
STERI/SOL mouthwash: lidocaine 1:1	

Oral Crust/Debris

Rinse with water qid until clear.

Hiccups

1 tsp white granulated sugar—swallowed dry

Medications to treat:

Baclofen *(Lioresal)*	10 mg po q 6h prn
Chlorpromazine *(Largactil)*	10–25 mg po/pr q 6h prn
Metoclopramide *(Maxeran)*	10 mg po/sc q 6h prn

Respiratory Symptoms

Dyspnea

- Treat underlying cause if able to do so
- Cool air, increase air circulation (open window, bedside fan)

Medications/treatments:
- Oxygen (use caution in COPD Patients)
- Opioid (e.g., oral or sc low-dose morphine; use hydromorphone or oxycodone in renal insufficiency); if currently on opioid, increase dose by 25–50%
- Anxiolytics:
  - Lorazepam 0.5–1 mg sl/sc q 1hr prn or regularly or
  - Midalzolam *(Versed)*: 0.5–1 mg sc q 10min followed by continuous infusion
- Steroid, e.g. dexamethasone *(Decadron)* 4 mg po/sc/iv bid-qid
- Ventolin 2.5 mg and atrovent 250 mcq (= 1 ml) N/S via nebulizer q 4h prn
- Other bronchodilators or diuretics as indicated
- Lasix can give 20 mg sc per site and/or atropine if congestion
- Radiotherapy

- Thoracentesis/pleuradesis, if collections of fluid in thoracic cavity-pleural effusion

Terminal Airway Secretions—"Death Rattle"

- Due to weakness, patient unable to clear secretions
- Suction if required and effective

Medications to treat:

Scopolamine *(hyoscine)*	0.4 mg–0.6 mg sc q 4 hrs prn (can be given regularly); also TransdermV, 1 patch q 3 days behind ear
Atropine *(Bentylol, Buscopan, Formulex)*	0.3–0.6 mg sc q 4h
Glycopyrolate	0.2–0.4 mg sc q 4h Note: Glycopyrolate has a slower onset, lasts twice as long, is more potent, and has less cardiac effects than atropine

Malignant Bowel Obstruction: Medications to treat

Medication	Route	Dosage	Schedule	Comments
Anti-nausea				
Haloperidol (*Haldol*)	SC or PO	0.5–2mg	Up to q 1h prn	Adverse effects rare at low dose
Metoclopramide (*Maxeran*)	SC or PO	5–20 mg or 5–10 mg	qid q 1h prn to max 80 mg/d	For partial obstruction may cause colic. Do not use in complete bowel obstruction
Methotremeprazine (*Nozinan*)	SC or PO	5–25 mg	q 4h prn	Nausea with colic pain. Sedating
Anti-secretory				
Octreotide (*Sandostatin*)	SC	100 mg– 500 mg	q 8–12h or continuous infusion	dries up secretions in bowels
Anti-colic				
Scopolamine (*TransdermV*)	Transdermal	Patch	q 3 days	Behind ear
Anti-inflammatory				
Dexamethasone (*Decadron*)	SC or PO	4 mg	od to qid	Decreases edema around the tumour
Ranitidine	PO or SC	50 mg sc q 8h	150 mg po bid	Decreases gastric secretions
PPIs such as: Losec Pantaloc	PO	20 mg od 40 mg od		Decreases gastric secretions

Subcutaneous Injections

These may be used with some medications where po/pr/iv not practical. Use a 25-gauge short butterfly needle when repeated subcutaneous injections anticipated. The butterfly must be primed with medication injected. Cover the injection site with Opsite or Tegaderm. Use a maximum volume of each injection of 2 cc. Change the site of injections if red, bleeding, swollen, leaking or sore.

Steroid Equivalency Chart

Drug	Dosage (mg)	Route of Administration
Dexamethasone *(Decadron)*	0.75	SC/IV/PO
Prednisone	5	PO

Commonly Used Abbreviations

Acronym	Term
SC (sc)	Subcutaneous
PO (po)	Per os (oral)
SL (sl)	Sublingual
PR (pr)	Per rectum
IV (iv)	Intravenous
IM (im)	Intramuscular
SR (sr)	Sustained Release
XR (xr)	Extended Release
CR (cr)	Controlled Release
IR (ir)	Immediate Release
CSCI (csci)	Continuous Subcutaneous Infusion
od	Once daily
bid	Two times per day
tid	Three times per day
qid	Four times per day
PRN (prn)	As needed
qxh	q = every; x = number; h = hours; q 4h = every four hours
PCA (pca)	Patient Controlled Analgesia
hs	At bedtime
R_x	Prescription
P_x	Prognosis
T_x	Treatment

Glossary of Commonly Used Ethical Terms

Many issues that occur in late- and end-stage dementia have ethical implications. There may be discussions between patients, families, professional caregivers, and members of an ethics committee. It is therefore important to understand some of the terms that are commonly used during such very importation conversations, as they may have a powerful impact on understanding and ultimate decisions.

Advance-care planning: Includes making decisions about the type of personal care, including health care, living arrangements, food, clothing, hygiene, and safety, that you want to receive in the future. This can be done by preparing a power of attorney for personal care or health care power of attorney (the second term is commonly used in the United States), in which you name a substitute decision-maker and provide whatever information is believed to be pertinent for future decision-making.

Advance directive or living will: A written document in which you clearly specify treatment preferences and how medical decisions affecting you are to be made if you are unable to make them. It usually also authorizes a specific person (surrogate decision-maker or proxy) to make such decisions on your behalf when you are no longer able to because of mental incapacity.

Artificial nutrition and hydration: A form of life-sustaining treatment. A chemically balanced mix of nutrients and fluids provided by placing a tube directly into the stomach, the intestine, or a vein.

Autonomy: One of the foundational ethical principles that says each person should be involved in making personal choices and have his or her choices respected within the bounds of the law, institutional values, and policies, and the sensibilities of staff and other clients. Clients'/patients' wishes should be solicited whenever possible and will be an essential component of health care decision-making, care planning, and following instructions in an advanced directive/living will.

Beneficence: Another foundational principle of medical ethics. Each staff member is obliged to do "good" and to promote others' welfare and well-being in accordance with the health care professionals' code of ethics and professional duties and obligations.

Best interest standard: A judgment based on an idea of what would be most beneficial to a patient, usually pursued in the absence of a patient's expressed wishes.

Cardiopulmonary resuscitation (CPR): An emergency procedure consisting of external cardiac massage and artificial respiration; the first treatment for a person who has collapsed, has no pulse, and has stopped breathing. Attempts to restore circulation of the blood and prevent death or brain damage due to lack of oxygen.

Codes of conduct/ethics: see Professional code of ethics.

Competent (also referred to as capable): A legal concept that describes people who are able to make their own decisions. Minors are presumed to be incompetent, except under certain specified conditions. The corollary medical-ethical term is *decisional capacity.*

Distributive justice: One of the foundational ethical principles. It is concerned with the fair allocation of resources among all members of a target community. Fair allocation generally includes the total amount of goods to be distributed, the distributing procedure, the conceptual support for the procedure, and the pattern of distribution that results.

Duty: The special responsibility associated with a particular profession or occupation or societal role. Physicians, journalists, students, and parents all have special duties. The duty of an individual or group includes descriptions about how the duty makes the group different from other groups in the society. This is also a key term in Kantian ethics: We have a duty to abide by the moral law built into our minds. Compromises and little white lies are not permissible.

Ethical dilemma: A moral conflict that involves determining appropriate conduct when an individual faces conflicting professional values and responsibilities.

Ethicist: One whose judgment on ethics and ethical codes has come to be trusted by some community, and (importantly) is expressed in some way that makes it possible for others to mimic or approximate that judgment. Professional who is skilled in helping people make decisions about what is morally right and wrong.

Ethics committee: An interdisciplinary group that deals with conflicts of values in patient care in acute and long-term settings. Such committees discuss policy issues (for example, regarding withholding and withdrawing of life-sustaining treatments).

Euthanasia: The act of either permitting a person to die or intentionally ending a person's life; generally rooted in motives of mercy, beneficence, or respect for patient dignity.

Informed consent: The legal and ethical requirement that no significant medical procedure can be performed until the competent patient has been informed of the nature of the procedure, risks, and alternatives, as well as the prognosis if the procedure is not done. The patient must freely and voluntarily agree to have the procedure done.

Justice: Each person has a right to be treated fairly in the process of making decisions (procedural justice) or in the way limited resources are allocated (distributive justice). Procedural justice is reflected when all interested parties have an opportunity to be heard and all options are explored when making decisions. Distributive justice considers access to health care and social service resources based on the various components of need.

Life-sustaining treatments: Used to maintain life in circumstances where, without such treatments, life is likely to end, with the usual understanding that such treatments are often temporary in nature until a person recovers from a serious illness or until a decision is made about future treatments. Examples of life-sustaining treatment include, but are not limited to, mechanical ventilation, renal dialysis, chemotherapy, and the administration of artificial nutrition and hydration.

Nonmaleficence: Another foundational ethical principle. Health care professionals are obliged whenever possible to prevent or do no harm. Nonmaleficence is linked to beneficence when health care professionals are (1) not doing evil nor causing harm, (2) preventing evil or harm, or (3) removing evil or sources of harm and thereby promoting good.

Palliative care: Medical or comfort care that reduces the severity of a disease or slows its progress rather than providing a cure. For incurable diseases, in cases where the cure is not recommended due to other health concerns, and when the patient does not wish to pursue a cure, palliative care becomes the focus of treatment. Among other things, palliative care strives to accomplish the following: provide relief from pain and other distressing symptoms; affirm life and regard dying as a normal process; intend neither to hasten or postpone death; integrate the psychological and spiritual aspects of patient care; and offer a support system to help patients live as actively as possible until death.

Passive euthanasia: Intentionally allowing a person to die by withholding or withdrawing treatment or by permitting the disease process to progress without further intervention. It is sometimes difficult to differentiate the natural course of disease from an act whose purpose is to specifically and intentionally promote death.

Power of Attorney for Personal Care (term commonly used in Canada), or **Health Care Power of Attorney** (term commonly used in the United States): A document in which you name a person or more than one person to be responsible for making personal decisions on your behalf should you become incapable. The person named on the document is known as the Attorney for Personal Care. You can also provide written instructions about the type of personal care that is preferred or rejected at some point in time in the future, should incapacity occur. Decisions about life-sustaining treatments such as ventilators, intensive care, and intravenous and tube feeding may be included.

Principlism: An approach to ethical thinking established in the 1970s that approaches ethical issues through a number of principles that allow a deliberative approach to understanding and resolution. These four foundational principles include respect for autonomy, nonmaleficence, beneficence, and justice.

Professional code of ethics: Professions are powerful social groups that have been assigned the responsibility to use their power for the good of the less powerful. A code of ethics is a formal statement that both claims that responsibility and gives guidance to its accomplishment. A code of ethics guides the responsible action of the professional.

Professional values (or duties): All health care professional groups have identified a set of expectations for each of their members. These expectations are based on what the professional group has agreed are the most important values, or virtues, to be maintained. Integrity, respect, and compassion are commonly cited as virtues expected of health care professionals.

Quality of life: Often contrasted with quantity or sanctity of life and indicates

146

that there are moral limits to the use of life-prolonging medical interventions. Quality of life is regarded as a patient-centered moral criterion, emphasizing the worth of the patient's own life to himself or herself.

Substituted judgment: A process whereby a proxy makes a decision about medical treatment for an incompetent patient based on his or her understanding of what the patient would have decided if competent. The substituted judgment standard has been important in influential legal decisions and is typically contrasted with the *best interest* standard.

Surrogate decision maker: A person or persons who will make decisions on behalf of an incapable person. Persons who are incapable are not able to understand the nature of treatment choices or appreciate the consequences of their decisions.

Ventilator: A breathing machine that is used to treat respiratory failure by promoting ventilation; also called a respirator.

Veracity: Each person is entitled to be told the truth, to the extent he or she wishes to know it. Caregivers expect truthful and accurate information from clients and their families. A relationship based on truth and sharing information in an objective, accurate, and comprehensive manner fosters trust among clients, their families, and health care professionals. This mutual trust is the essential element in relationships formed to meet the common goal of enriching the quality of life of the client and providing the highest quality of care.

Vulnerable patient (or person): Vulnerable means wounded and unable to defend oneself. Patients have a strong self-perception of vulnerability, but truly vulnerable patients are those who cannot act on their own to protect themselves from threats to their health and dignity. Vulnerable patients are powerless.

References and Further Reading

1. Alzheimer Society of Canada. *History Highlights*, cited September 2008. http://www.alzheimer.ca/english/society/history-highlights.htm.

2. Brooker, D., Edwards P., and Benson, S., eds. *DCM Experience and Insights into Practice*. Hawker Publications: London, 2004.

3. Buchman, D., Buchman, S., Grossman, D., Caratao, R., and Kirstein, A. Baycrest Geriatric Health Care System Palliative Care Handbook. Toronto, 2005.

4. Clark, D. "Between Hope and Acceptance: the Medicalisation of Dying." *BMJ* (2002): 324:905–907.

5. Collier, J., and Iheanacho, I. "The Pharmaceutical Industry as an Informant." *Lancet* (2002): 360:1405–9.

6. Doyle, D., Hanks, G., Cherny, N.I., and Calman, K., eds. *Oxford Textbook of Palliative Medicine*. New York: Oxford University Press, 2003.

7. Evers, et al. "Palliative and Aggressive End-of-Life Care for Patients with Dementia." *Psychiatric Services* (2002): 53:609–613.

8. Finucane T.E., Christmas, C., and Travis K. "Palliative and Aggressive End-of-Life Care for Patients with Dementia." *JAMA* (1999): 282:1365–1370.

9. Gillick, M.R., and Mitchell, S.L.214969 "Facing Eating Difficulties in End-Stage Dementia." *Alzheimer's Care Quarterly* (2002): 3:227–232.

10. Gordon, M. "CPR in Long-Term Care: Mythical Benefits or Necessary Ritual." *Annals of Long-Term Care: Clinical Care and Aging* (2003): 11:41–49.

11. Hughes, J.C., Robinson, L., and Volicer, L., "Specialist Palliative Care in Dementia." *BMJ* (2005): 330:57–58.

12. Hughes, J., Jolley, D., Jordan, A., and Sampson E., "Palliative Care in Dementia: Issues and Evidence." *Advances in Psychiatric Treatment* (2007) 134:251–260.

13. Hurley, A.C., Volicer, B.J., and Volicer, L.: "Effect of Fever Management Strategy on the Progress of Dementia of the Alzheimer Type." *Alzheimer Disease and Associated Disorders* (1996): 10:5–10.

14. Jennings, S. *Creative Play and Drama with Adults at Risk.* Speechmark: Bicester, 2004.

15. Koopmans, R.T.C.M., Pasman, H.R. , and van der Steen, J.T. "Palliative Care in Patients with Severe Dementia." In A. Burns and B. Winblad, eds., *Severe Dementia,* pp. 205–213. London: John Wiley & Sons, Ltd., 2006.

16. Librach, L.S., and Squires, B.P. . *The Pain Manual: Principles and Issues in Cancer Pain Management,* Pegasus Healthcare International: Toronto, 1997.

17. Mitchell et al. "The Clinical Course of Advanced Dementia." *New England Journal of Medicine* (2009): 361:1529–1538.

18. Morrison, R.S., and Siu, A.L. . "Survival in End-Stage Dementia Following Acute Illness." *JAMA* (2000): 284:47–52.

19. Moss et al. "The Metaphor of 'Family' in Staff Communication about Dying and Death." *Journal of Gerontology, Series B: Psychological Sciences and Social Sciences* (2003): 58:290.

20. Nolan et al. "Beyond 'Person-Centred' Care: a New Vision for Gerontological Nursing." *International Journal of Older People Nursing* (2004): 13:45–53.

21. Sachs, G.A., Shega, J.W. , and Cox-Hayley, D. . "Barriers to Excellent End-of-Life Care for Patients with Dementia." *Journal of General Internal Medicine* (2004): 19:1057–1063.

22. Sabat, S.R. *The Experience of Alzheimer's Disease: Life through a Tangled Veil.* Oxford, U.K.: Blackwell Publishers, 2001.

23. Solomon, S. "End-of-Life War Outlives Golubchuck." *National Review of Medicine,* July 2008, Volume 5, number 7. http://www.nationalreviewofmedicine.com/issue/2008/07/5_patients_practice_07.html.

24. Statistics Canada. *Population projections for 2001, 2006, 2011, 2016, 2021, and 2026.* July 1. [cited February 11, 2002]. http://www.statcan.ca/english/Pgdb/People/Population/demo23b.htm.

25. Volicer, L., et al. "Characteristics of Dementia End-of-Life Care Across Care Settings." *American Journal of Hospital Palliative Care* (2003): 20:191–200.

26. Volicer, L. *End-of-Life Care for People with Dementia in Residential Care Settings.* Alzheimer's Association, 2005.

Resources

The Rising Tide Study—A report released by The Alzheimer Society of Canada with information about the projected economic and social costs of dementia.
http://www.alzheimer.ca/docs/RisingTide/Rising%20Tide_Full%20 Report_Eng_FINAL_Secured%20version.pdf.

Progression Series and Physician's Corner of the Alzheimer Society of Canada
http://www.Alzheimer.ca (look under Alzheimer's disease: Progression of Alzheimer's Disease (stages) and Physician's Corner)

The IAHPC Manual of Palliative Care 2nd Edition
http://www.hospicecare.com/manual/toc-main.html

A Caregiver's Guide Handbook about End-of-Life Care—Developed in 2000 by the Edmonton Commandery in association with the Palliative Care Association of Alberta, the Alberta Cancer Board, and the Edmonton Regional Palliative Care Program.
http://www.stlazarus.ca/english/news_pages/caregiversguide.html

End-of-Life Care for Seniors: A Comprehensive Approach
http://seniorcarecanada.com/articles/2001/q3/end.of.life/

A Guide for Caregivers: Living lessons—An innovative program developed by The GlaxoSmithKline Foundation in partnership with the Canadian Hospice Palliative Care Association (CHPCA).
http://www.chpca.net/resource_doc_library/caregiver_resource_ inventory/20-Living_%20Lessons-AGuideforCaregivers.pdf

Caregiver, Patient, and Physician Resources for the Hospice Palliative Care Community
http://www.living-lessons.org/resources/secured/resources_home.asp

Cross-Cultural Considerations in Promoting Advance Care Planning in Canada—Developed by the Palliative and End-of-Life Care Unit, Chronic and Continuing Care Division, Secretariat on Palliative and End-of-Life Care, Primary and Continuing Health Care Division of the Health Care Policy Directorate, Health Canada.
http://www.bccancer.bc.ca/NR/rdonlyres/E17D408A-C0DB-40FA-9682-9DD914BB771F/28582/COLOUR030408_Con.pdf

The Ontario government "Life Event" bundle—Information and resources for finding end-of-life care.
http://www.ontario.ca/en/life_events/senior/004539

A toolkit of instruments to measure end-of-life care from Brown University
http://www.chcr.brown.edu/pcoc/TOOLKIT.htm

Educational materials from End-of-life/Palliative Education Resource Center-Medical College of Wisconsin
http://www.eperc.mcw.edu/EPERC/EducationalMaterials

Articles on palliative care education from End-of-life/Palliative Education Resource Center, Medical College of Wisconsin
http://www.eperc.mcw.edu/EPERC/WhatsNew/Articles

Ian Anderson Continuing Education Program in End-of-Life care, University of Toronto
http://www.cepd.utoronto.ca/endoflife/

Index

A

abbreviations, commonly used, 142

acetaminophen (Acet), 113, 114, 115, 120

acid reflux, 89, 98, 99–100

activities of daily living (ADLs), 6

acupuncture, 77, 81, 95, 120

acute constipation, 81

Adamson, Lynn J., 10

addiction to medications, fear of, 70

adhesive films, 106

adjuvants, 113, 117, 120, 124

ADLs (activities of daily living), 6

advance directive, 30, 31, 63, 65, 143

advance-care planning, 143

agitation
    approaches/interventions for, 93
    as nonverbal cue, 60

alcohol abuse, effect of, 5

Alertec (modafinil), 74, 75, 79, 80

Alzheimer Association (US), 3

Alzheimer Society of Canada, 3, 149

Alzheimer's Association, 14

Alzheimer's disease
    as leading form of dementia, 4
    progression of, 11–12
    as terminal disease, 11, 12

amantadine, 93

amitriptyline, 73, 115, 124

analgesics, 39, 105, 107, 111, 113, 115, 117, 120, 123, 125

anal/rectal pathology, 82

anesthetics, local, 120

anhedonia, 71

anorexia
    approaches/interventions for, 79–81
    causes of, 78
    clinical presentation of, 77, 78

anorexia-cachexia syndrome, 78

antacids, 86, 99–100, 138

anticholinergic agents, 89, 90, 93, 98, 99

anticholinergic effects, 82, 115, 124

anticonvulsants, 120

antidepressants, 5, 73, 120

anti-emetics, 126

antifungals, azole antifungals, 101

antihistamines, 90, 130

anti-inflammatory medications, 125

antineoplastics, 98

antipsychotics, 77, 90, 136

antispasmodics, 120

anxiety
    approaches/interventions for, 76–77
    causes of, 76
    clinical presentation of, 75

anxiolytics, 139

aphtlous ulcers, 102

Arelia (pamidronate), 124
aromatherapy, 77, 94, 95, 105
art therapy, 70, 76, 117, 120
arthritic pain, 114
arthritis, and dementia, 17, 59
artificial hydration, 36, 38, 143, 145. *see also* hydration
artificial nutrition, 36, 38, 143, 145. *see also* nutrition
ASA, 89
aspiration pneumonia, 5, 6, 36
Ativan (lorazepam), 76, 93, 97, 128, 135, 136, 139
atropine (Bentylol, Buscopan, Formulex), 97, 102, 139, 140
atrovent, 139
atypical antipsychotics, 90
atypical neuroleptics, 5
autonomy, 26, 48, 57–61, 143–144
azole antifungals, 101

B

baclofen (Lioresal), 139
bedsores, 102
behavioural cues, 60
beneficence, as ethical principle of care, 26, 144
Bentylol (atropine), 97, 102, 139, 140
benzodiazepines, 76, 77, 92, 93, 97, 99, 136
benzydamine HCl (Tantum), 138
bereavement
    before actual death of loved one, 52
    and depression in patient, 71, 72
    of patient, approaches/interventions for, 72
best interest standard, 144
biochemical disorders, and nausea/vomiting, 89
biofeedback, 77

biotene gel, 110, 137
biphosphanates, 99
bisacodyl (Dulcolax), 86–87, 127
bisphosphonates, 116, 120, 124
body language
    from health care professionals, 56
    of patients, 59
bone pain, 116–117, 124
Bonefos (clodronate), 124
bowel obstruction (malignant), medications to treat, 141
Braden, B., 107
brain exercises, as risk reducer, 4
"breakthrough" pain medication, 123–124
breathing exercises, 76
breathlessness
    approaches/interventions for, 95
    causes of, 94–95
    clinical presentation of, 94
bronchodilators, 139
bronchospasms, 95
Brooker, D., 57, 149
bulk-forming agents, for constipation treatment, 83
Buscopan (atropine), 97, 102, 139, 140
butyrophenones, 90

C

cachexia (wasting)
    approaches/interventions for, 78–81
    causes of, 78
    clinical presentation of, 77–78
calcitonin, 117
calcium, 82
calcium channel blockers, 99
calmness, from health care professionals, 56
camphor, 130
Canada

as cultural mosaic, 45
statistics on age of population, 3
Canadian Medical Association, 69
Canadian Palliative Care Association, 16
cancer care, 16
CancerCare Ontario (CCO), 16, 17
cannabinoids, 91, 125
capable, defined, 144
capacity, of patient to make informed decisions, 29–30
capsaicin, 116
carbamazepine (Tegretol), 125
cardiac disease, 78. *see also* heart disease
cardiopulmonary resuscitation (CPR), 20, 40–41, 42, 144
cardiovascular disease, 76. *see also* heart disease
caregiver burden, 49
caregivers
caring for, 49–56
impacts of being, 50
caregiving
challenges and benefits of, 56
process of, 51–52
cascara sagrada, 85–86
CCO (CancerCare Ontario), 16, 17
central nervous system disturbances, and nausea/vomiting, 89, 90
Cephlac (lactulose), 86, 127
chaplains, 69
chemical disorders, and nausea/vomiting, 89
chemotherapy
as cause of nausea/vomiting, 89
for controlling tumour growth, 105
as life-sustaining treatment, 17, 145
palliative chemotherapy, 117, 120
chest physiotherapy, 96
Cheyne-Stokes breathing, 97
Chinese medicine, traditional, 81

chlordiazepoxide, 77
chlorpromazine (Largactil), 97, 126, 135, 139
cholestyramine (Questran), 130
chronic constipation, 81
chronic disease, 11
chronic pain, and anxiety, 76
chronic wounds
approaches/interventions for, 104–108
causes of, 103–104
clinical presentation of, 102–103
Chronulac (lactulose), 86, 127
cimetidine, 100
clinical depression
approaches/interventions for, 73
as differentiated from sadness, 72
clodronate (Bonefos), 124
clonazepam (Rivotril), 125, 128
clostridium difficile, 35
clozapine, 94
code of ethics, 146
codeine, 96, 113, 114, 115, 120, 121, 122, 123
cognitive behavior therapy, as non-pharmacologic adjuvant, 120
coherence, patient's lack of, 57
Colace (docusate), 127
comfort, as palliative care priority, 20
communication
about bad news, 29
about end-of-life decisions, 25, 27–28, 40
as conflict-prevention strategy, 42
cultural implications of, 48
family members as main avenue of, 34
importance of, 40, 59, 118
lack of, 8, 9
patient's decreased ability for, 59
co-morbid conditions, 15, 59, 76, 78

compassion, from health care professionals, 56

competent, defined, 144

complementary therapies
for anxiety, 77
and culture traditions, 48
for depression, 75
for dyspnea/breathlessness/respiratory problems, 95
for hallucinations/perceptual disturbances, 94
inquiry about in assessments, 69
for pain relief/management, 117, 120
for weight loss/anorexia/cachexia, 81

confidentiality
acceptability of breaching of, 35
methods to assure protection of, 34

conflict
among family members, 62–65
dealing with, 41–42

connecting, finding different ways of, 54–55

consent
implied consent, 35
informed consent, 28–29, 145
test of, 35

consent, test of, 35

constipation
anal/rectal pathology, 82
approaches/interventions for, 83
causes of, 81–82
clinical presentation of, 81
concurrent disease states, 82
medications for, 82
as side effect of opioids, 85, 88, 115, 127

control model, 5

COPD, and anorexia-cachexia syndrome, 78

cord compression, 137–138

Cornell Scale for Depression in Dementia, 72

corticosteroids, 99, 120

cough assist device, 96

cough suppressants, 96

coughs, 95

counseling, as non-pharmacologic adjuvant, 120

COX-2 specific NSAIDs, 114–115, 116, 124

CPR (cardiopulmonary resuscitation), 20, 40–41, 42, 144

crossword puzzles, as risk reducer, 4

cultural implications, 37, 38, 41, 45–48

curative model, 5

cyclic drugs, 124

cyclizine, 90

cyclokapron, 105

cytoprotective agents, 114

Cytotec (misoprostol), 114

D

death
context of, 7–8
cultural impact on understandings and rituals of, 45
medicalization of, 8, 9

"death rattle," 140

Decadron (dexamethasone), 74, 79, 80, 96, 116, 125, 130, 136, 137, 139, 141, 142

decisional capacity, 144

decision-making process
and artificial feeding, 13, 36
"do not resuscitate" option, 41
ethical approach to, 46
as guided by patient's values, beliefs, culture, 41
how to avoid conflicts in, 63
impact of ethno-cultural beliefs on, 47–48
impact of religious perspectives on, 8, 47–48

as ongoing, 27
overview of, 32
and palliative care, 20–21
patient's participation in, 12, 26, 28–29, 30, 35, 144
potential difficulties with, 7
as shared, 29, 31, 40, 42, 48, 51–52
decubitus ulcers, 102
dehydration
  approaches/interventions for, 109–110
  causes of, 108
  clinical presentation of, 108
delirium
  and anorexia-cachexia syndrome, 78
  and anxiety, 76
  approaches/interventions for, 92–94
  causes of, 92
  clinical presentation of, 91
  as side effect of opioids, 135
dementia
  and anorexia-cachexia syndrome, 78
  and anxiety, 76
  average length of end stages of, 7
  clinical course of, 14–15
  and delirium, 91, 92
  length of, compared to other fatal illnesses, 10
  overview of, 4–5, 13
  as process that has no end, 8
  progression of, 17
  risk factors for, 4
  statistics on likelihood of having, 54
denial
  of family members about dementia, 52
  as reaction to diagnosis, 8
dental hygiene, 101. see also mouth care
Depakene, 125
depression
  and anxiety, 76
  approaches/interventions for, 72–74
  clinical presentation of, 71
desipramine, 73, 102, 115

dexamethasone (Decadron), 74, 79, 80, 96, 116, 125, 130, 136, 137, 139, 141, 142
dextromethorphan, 96
diabetes, and dementia, 17
diabetes mellitus, as risk factor for dementia, 4
diazepam (Valium), 77, 128, 136
diet, as risk factor for dementia, 4
dietary requirements, cultural implications of, 48
dieticians, 79
Diflucan (fluconazole), 101, 138
dihydropyridines, 99
Dilantin, 136
dimenhydrinate (Gravol), 90, 126
disagreements, among family members, 63
disbelief, as reaction to diagnosis, 8
disclosure, of information, 29
disenfranchised grief, 55
distributive justice, 144, 145
diuretics, 139
do not resuscitate order (DNR order), 41
docusate (Colace), 127
docusate calcium, 83
docusate sodium, 83
domperidone (Motilium), 88, 91, 100, 127
donut-type devices, 107
dopamine agents, 93
dosing
  Opioid Dosing table, 121–122
  prn dosing, 117
  round-the-clock dosing, 117
doxepin (Sinequan), 73, 130
doxycycline, 99
doxycycline pleurodesis, 96
Dr. Gordon Discusses
  advance directives, 64

consequences of lack of communication, 27–28
decision-making process, 32–34
dementia, natural outcome of, 15
feeding tube, 37–39
feelings of family members, 53–54
parent adamant about not leaving home, 50–51
patient's decreased ability to communicate, 59–60
quantity of life vs. quality of life, 6–7
Samuel Golubchuk story, 18–20
terminal diseases, 11–12
working with Jewish family, 46–47
drugs, recreational, 5
dry mouth, 98, 102, 137–138. *see also* dehydration
dry mucous membranes, 110
Dulcolax (bisacodyl), 86–87, 127
duty, as ethical term, 144
dysesthetic pain, 112, 115
dysphagia
approaches/interventions for, 99–102
causes of, 98
clinical presentation of, 97–98
dyspnea (shortness of breath)
and anxiety, 76
approaches/interventions for, 95
causes of, 94–95
clinical presentation of, 94
as side effect of opioids, 139

E

eating. *see* diet; feeding techniques; feeding tubes; nutrition; tube feeding
eating skills, 98
edema (fluid retention), 38
education
on analgesic needs of patient, 117
of families, 61
of professionals, 60–61
of the public, 60

electrolyte disturbances, 89
emotional agitation, as nonverbal cue, 60
empathy, from health care professionals, 56
end of life, through different cultural lenses, 45–48
end-of-life care
compared to palliative care, 17, 110
improvements in, 20–21
nutrition and hydration in, 35
as subset of palliative care, 16
trends in, 14
end-of-life decision making. *see* decision-making process
end-of-life decisions, communication about, 25, 27–28, 40
end-of-life issues, recent spotlight on, 3
end-of-life symptoms, 77
enemas, 87, 127
environmental irritants, 95
epidural, 125
Epival, 125
Equianalgesic Chart, 122–123
esophageal candidiasis, 101
esophageal ulcers, 100
ethical dilemmas, 144
ethical issues, of patient care, 39
ethical principles, of patient care, 25–27, 42, 144, 145
ethical terms, glossary of, 143–147
ethicists, 40, 42, 63, 64, 144–145
ethics, code of, 146
ethics committees, 145
ethno-cultural-religious gaps, 47, 48
ethno-cultural-religious views, 37, 38
euthanasia, 18, 19, 145. *see also* passive euthanasia
excessive salivation, 102
exercise, lack of, as risk factor for dementia, 4

exercise program, 115

The Experience of Alzheimer's Disease: Life Through a Tangled Veil (Sabat), 58

eye contact, from health care professionals, 56

F

facial expressions
  of health care professionals, 56
  as nonverbal cues, 60
family conflict, 62–65
family members
  conflict among, 62–65
  feelings of, 52, 53–54
  importance of routine for, 52
  as main avenue of communication, 34
  suffering of, 56
family unit, and culture, 48
famotidine, 100
fear, and reluctance to report symptoms, 68
fecal impaction, 81, 84, 85, 87–88, 89
feeding techniques, 38, 101
feeding tubes, 12, 31, 32–33, 36, 37–38. *see also* tube feeding
fentanyl, 107, 113, 120, 122, 123
fibre content, 83
Finucane, T. E., 17, 149
flax, 83
Fleet Enema, 127
fluconazole (Diflucan), 101, 138
fluid restrictions, 96
fluid retention (edema), 38
flurazepam, 77
Formulex (atropine), 97, 102, 139, 140
Fowler's Position, 95
fungating lesion, 103
furosemide, 96

G

gabapentin (Neurontin), 116, 125
gastrostomy tube (G-tube), 37
gender roles, cultural implications of, 48
Geriatric Depression Scale, 72
Gillick, M. R., 38, 149
Global Deterioration Scale, 7
glycerin suppositories, 86, 88, 127
glycerin swabs, 110, 137
glycopyrrolate, 97, 102, 140
Golubchuk, Samuel, 18–19
Gravol (dimenhydrinate), 90, 126
grief
  before actual death of loved one, 52
  coping with, 55–56
  cultural implications of, 48
G-tube (gastrostomy tube), 37

H

H2 antagonists (Zantac), 91, 100, 101
HADS (Hospital Anxiety and Depression Scale), 72
hallucinations/perceptual disturbances, approaches/interventions for, 93
haloperidol (Haldol), 90, 93, 126, 135, 141
hand-feeding, 38
hands-on training, for care providers, 60
Harvard University, 14, 37, 38
Health Canada, 122
Health Care Consent Act (1996) (Ontario), 28, 30
health care professionals
  body language of, 56
  calmness from, 56
  compassion from, 56
  coping with grief, 55–56
  empathy from, 56
  eye contact from, 56
  facial expressions of, 56

hugs from, 56
  narrative work of, 58
  values and duties of, 146
  voice of, 56
hearing, as way of connecting to loved
  one, 55
heart disease, 17, 59. *see also* cardiac
  disease; cardiovascular disease
hiccups, 139
high blood pressure, as risk factor for
  dementia, 4
homeopathy, 75, 94
Hospital Anxiety and Depression Scale
  (HADS), 72
hospital ethicist, 40. *see also* ethicists
hugs from, from health care professionals, 56
humidifier, 138
hunger, 37
hydration, 35–36, 42. *see also* artificial
  hydration
hydrocodone, 96
hydrocolloids, 106
hydromorphone, 96, 113, 115, 120,
  121, 122, 123, 126, 139
hyoscine (scolopamine), 140
hyoscine butylbromide, 90
hyoscine hydrobromide, 97
hypercalcemia, 82, 89, 92, 135
hyperlipidemia (elevated or abnormal
  blood fats), as risk factor for dementia,
  4
hypertension (high blood pressure), as
  risk factor for dementia, 4
hyperthyroidism, and anorexia-cachexia
  syndrome, 78
hypodermoclysis, 109
hyponatremia, 73, 92, 109
hypotension, 73, 94
hypoxia, 96, 135

I

IM route, 126
imipramine, 73
implied consent, 35
inanition, 37
influenza infections, 35
information disclosure, 29
informed consent, 28–29, 145
intestinal tract motility, 88
intramuscular injections, cautions with,
  117
intravenous therapy, 17, 38
ipratropium bromide, 95
iron, 82
itraconazole, 101

J

Jennings, S., 57, 150
Judaism, perspectives on life and death,
  19, 46–47
justice, as ethical principle of care,
  26–27, 145

K

Kantian ethics, 144
ketoconazole (Nizoral), 100, 101, 138
ketocozole, 101
ketones, 37

L

laboratory tests, as intervention, 17
lactulose (Chronulate, Cephlac), 86,
  127
lansoprazole, 100
Largactil (chlorpromazine), 97, 126,
  135, 139
Lasix, 139

Lax-a-day, 85, 127

laxatives, 127

legal intervention, 40

legal issues, 29, 35, 39, 40, 51, 144, 145, 147

legal services, for advance directive, 63

levodopa preparations, 93

Lewy Body dementia, 99

lidocaine, 102, 138

life history reviews, 58

life passages, cultural impact on, 45

life-support
    discomfort of, 19–20
    discontinuance of, 19
    and Samuel Golubchuk story, 18, 19
    standard for, 19

life-sustaining treatments
    defined, 145
    withholding or stopping of, 40–41

lifting devices, 107

Lioresal (baclofen), 139

living will, 63, 64, 65, 143

long-term care, average length of, 3–4

long-term care facilities
    moving parent to, 50–51
    and participation of family members in care, 52

lorazepam (Ativan), 76, 93, 97, 128, 135, 136, 139

Losec, 141

loss, before actual death of loved one, 52

Lyrica (pregabalin), 116, 125

M

Maalox, 138

magnesium hydroxide (MOM), 84, 85–86

malignancy, and anorexia-cachexia syndrome, 78

malignant obstruction, and dyspnea/breathlessness/respiratory problems, 96

malnutrition, 77–78

massage therapy, 54, 69, 70, 76, 94, 120

mattresses, 104, 107, 131

Maxeran (metoclopramide), 88, 91, 99, 100, 126, 127, 139, 141

mechanical obstruction, 88–89

mechanical ventilation, 145

meclizine, 90

mediator, 42

medical ethicist, 42. *see also* ethicists

medications. *see also* analgesics; antidepressants; *specific medications*
    behaviour-modifying, 5
    for bone pain, 124
    "breakthrough" pain medication, 123–124
    for constipation, 82, 127
    for delirium, 135
    fear of addiction to, 70
    for hiccups, 139
    for myoclonic jerks, 128
    for neuropathic pain, 125
    for oral candidiasis, 138
    over-the-counter, 69
    for pain relief, 39
    principles for use of, 69–70
    prn dosing, 117
    reluctance to take, 70
    "rescue" medication, 123–124
    for respiratory depression, 128–130
    for restlessness, 135
    round-the-clock dosing, 117
    for seizures, 136
    for skin breakdown, 135
    for skin care, 130
    for terminal airway secretions/"death rattle," 140
    for ulceration and stomatitis, 138–139

and weight loss, 79

megace (megestrol) acetate, 79, 80

menthol, 130

methadone, 113, 116, 125

methicillin-resistant staphylococcus aureus (MRSA), 35

methotrimeprazine (Nozinan), 90, 93, 126, 135, 141

methylnaltrexone (Relistor), 88, 127

methylphenidate (Ritalin), 74–75, 79, 80

metoclopramide (Maxeran), 88, 91, 99, 100, 126, 127, 139, 141

metronidazole, 105, 135

midazolam (Versed), 97, 105, 128, 135, 136, 139

mineral oil, 84, 87

MiraLAX, 85, 127

mirtazapine (Remeron), 130

misoprostol (Cytotec), 114

Mitchell, Susan L., 14, 15, 17, 37, 38, 150

modafinil (Alertec), 74, 75, 79, 80

moisturizers, 108, 130

MOM (magnesium hydroxide), 84, 85–86

morphine, 96, 105, 115, 120, 121, 122, 123, 126, 139

Moss, M. S., 55

motility agents, 127

Motilium (domperidone), 88, 91, 100, 127

mourning, cultural implications of, 48

mouth care, 38, 98, 101, 110, 137

mouth rinse, 102

move to care facility, patients' resistance to, 51

MRSA (methicillin-resistant staphylococcus aureus), 35

mucosal irritation, 89

music, value of, 55

music therapy, 70, 76, 94, 117, 120

mycostatin (Nystatin), 100, 138

myoclonic jerks, as side effect of opioids, 128

N

nabilone, 91

naloxone (Narcan), 128–130

narcotics, 9, 107

narrative work, of health care professionals, 58

National Pressure Ulcer Advisor Panel, 104

nature images, value of, 55

nausea
    approaches/interventions for, 90
    causes of, 89
    clinical presentation of, 88
    as side effect of opioids, 89, 126

nerve block, 125

neuralgic pain, 112

neuroleptics, 5, 82, 93, 99

neurological symptoms, as side effect of opioids, 135

Neurontin (gabapentin), 116, 125

neuropathic pain, 74, 112, 115–116, 125

neuropathy, peripheral, 59

neuro-vegetative symptoms, 72

nitrates, 99

Nizoral (ketoconazole), 100, 101, 138

nociceptive pain, 112

Nolan, M.R., 59

non-maleficence, as ethical principle of care, 26, 145

non-medicinal approaches, 69

nonopioid analgesics, 113

non-pharmacologic therapy, 5, 70, 76, 83, 91, 117, 118, 120

non-traditional practitioners, 69

nonverbal cues, 59–60, 68

Non-Verbal Depression Scale, 72

Norton, D., 107

nortriptyline, 73, 102, 115, 124

Nozinan (methotrimeprazine), 90, 93, 126, 135, 141

NSAIDs, 89, 114, 116, 120, 124

nutrition, as ethical dilemma, 35–36

Nystatin (mycostatin), 100, 138

O

occupational therapy, 70, 107

octreotide (Sandostatin), 91, 141

olanzapine (Zyprexa), 79, 80, 90, 93, 94, 135

omeprazole, 100

Opioid Dosing Table, 121–122

opioid naïve, 96, 105, 120, 122

opioids

    controlling side effects of, 126

    side effects of, 83, 85, 89, 90, 126, 127, 128–129, 135, 136, 138, 139–140

    use of, 70, 76, 82, 89, 96, 97, 98, 99, 115, 117, 120, 121–123, 124, 128, 129, 135, 139

oral candidiasis, 100, 138

oral complications

    approaches/interventions for, 99–102

    causes of, 98

    clinical presentation of, 97–98

oral crust/debris, 139

oral lesions, 98

osmotic agents, for constipation treatment, 86

osteoporosis, and dementia, 59

oxazepam, 76

Oxford Textbook of Palliative Medicine, 49

oxycocet, 122

oxycodone, 96, 113, 115, 120, 122, 123, 139

OxyContin, 122, 123

oxygen, 139

P

pain

    approaches/interventions for, 39, 113–118, 123–125

    arthritic pain, 114

    assessment of, 113

    bone pain, 116–117, 124

    causes of, 112–113

    chronic pain, 76

    clinical presentation of, 110–111

    dysesthetic pain, 112, 115

    neuralgic pain, 112

    neuropathic pain, 74, 112, 115–116, 125

    nociceptive pain, 112

    relief of, 39–40

pain assessment, and wound procedures, 106

pain management, 120

palliative care

    compared to end-of-life care, 17, 110

    described, 6, 9, 15–18, 20, 48, 59, 118, 145–146

    having discussions about, 25, 28, 32

    increased interest in, 61

    and individuality of each patient, 45

    and IV access, 136

    as likely choice, 32

    main goal of, 39

    and nutrition/hydration, 35, 109

    pain assessment scales, 119–120

    and person-centered approach, 61

Palliative Care Handbook (Grossman et al.), 121

pamidronate (Arelia), 124

Pantaloc, 141

pantoprazole, 100

Parkinson's disease
   and anorexia-cachexia syndrome, 78
   and depression, 71
   and dysphagia/oral complications, 99
   and hallucinations, 93, 94
   and skin breakdown/chronic
     wounds, 104
paroxetine, 130
passive euthanasia, 146
patients
   and bereavement, 71, 72
   body language of, 59
   capacity to make informed decisions,
     29–30
   decreased ability for communication,
     59
   importance of support for, 21
   lack of personal coherence, 57
   lack of verbal expression of, 58
   participation in decision-making
     process, 12, 26, 28–29, 30, 35, 144
   perspective of, taking consideration
     of, 26, 45, 57–59, 61
   treatment of, as individuals, 58
   views on suffering, 28, 35
   vulnerability of, 147
   wishes and values, 41, 63. *see also*
     advance directive
PEG procedure (percutaneous endoscopic gastrostomy), 37, 83, 85, 88
penicillin, 138
peripheral neuropathy, and dementia,
   59
personal coherence, patient's lack of, 57
person-centered care
   cultural implications of, 48
   and palliative care approach, 61
   principles of, 57–59, 147
petroleum jelly, 110, 138
pharmaceutical industry, financial
   interests of, 3
phenobarbital, 136
phenothiazines, 90, 98, 99

physical agitation, as nonverbal cue, 60
physical touch, role of, 48
physiotherapy, 70, 96, 97, 107, 114,
   115, 117
pleuradesis, 140
pleural effusion, 96
pneumonia, aspiration pneumonia, 5,
   6, 35
polyethylene glycol, 85
potassium salts, 99
power of attorney, 143, 146
PPIs, 141
prednisone, 95, 142
pregabalin (Lyrica), 116, 125
pressure sores, 102–107
Prevacid, 91
pride
   cautions with, 54
   and reluctance to report symptoms,
     68
principlism, as ethical term, 146
privacy, 34–35, 48, 87, 127
prn dosing, 117
procedural justice, 145
prochlorperazine (Stemetil), 90, 126
professional awareness, need for, 60
prokinetic agents
   for constipation treatment, 88
   for dysphagia/oral complications,
     100
   for nausea/vomiting treatment, 91
propylene glycol, 127
proton pump inhibitors, 91, 100, 101,
   114
proxy decision-maker, 30. *see also* substitute decision-maker (SDM)
prunes/prune juice, 83, 88
pruritis, 130
psychoactive substances, 5
psychologists, 69

psychomotor retardation/somnolence, 74–75

psyllium, 83

public awareness, need for, 60

pulmonary edema, 95, 96, 108

PUSH tool, 104

Q

quality of life, 7, 15, 16, 17, 19, 20, 36, 37, 41, 47, 59, 61, 146–147

quantity of life, 7, 146

Questran (cholestyramine), 130

quetiapine (Seroquel), 93, 94, 135

R

radiation therapy, 17, 89, 120, 136

radiotherapy, 116, 117, 124, 139

ranitidine, 100, 114, 141

Reagan, Ronald, 54

Red River Cereal, 83

relaxation techniques, 70, 76, 95, 117, 120

religious perspectives, 7, 8, 19, 26, 31, 33, 37, 38, 39, 41, 45, 46, 47–48

Relistor (methylnaltrexone), 88, 127

Remeron (mirtazapine), 130

renal dialysis, 145

repositioning
  cautions with, 106
  recommendations for, 107

"rescue" medication, 123

respectfulness, 26, 28, 29, 31, 34, 41, 42, 45, 46, 51, 57, 64, 73, 143, 145, 146

respiratory depression, as side effect of opioids, 128–129

respiratory problems
  approaches/interventions for, 95

causes of, 94–95
clinical presentation of, 94

respiratory symptoms, as side effect of opioids, 128, 139–140

restlessness
  approaches/interventions for, 93
  as side effect of opioids, 135

RestoraLAX, 85, 127

restraint, as intervention, 17

the "right" decision, 47

risperidone (Risperdal), 90, 93, 135

Ritalin (methylphenidate), 74–75, 79, 80

Rivotril (clonazepam), 125, 128

role playing, for care providers, 60

round-the-clock dosing, 117

routine, importance of establishing for family members, 52

S

Sabat, Steven R., 58

Sachs, Greg A., 18

sadness, 71, 72–73

salbutamol, 95

saline
  for constipation, 84
  for dehydration, 109
  for dry mouth, 138
  for dysphagia/oral complications, 102
  for dyspnea/breathlessness/respiratory problems, 95, 97
  for respiratory depression, 129
  for skin breakdown/chronic wounds, 104, 105, 131, 132, 133, 134
  for ulceration and stomatitis, 138

salivation, excessive, 102

salt restrictions, 96

sanctity of life, as theme of monotheistic religions, 47

Sandostatin (octreotide), 91, 141

Sativex spray, 116, 125

scales, for pain assessment, 119–120

scolopamine, 90, 97, 102

scolopamine (hyoscine), 140

scolopamine (TransdermV), 141

SDM (substitute decision-maker), 26, 29, 30–31, 38, 39–40, 47, 63, 143

second guessing, cautions with, 47

secretions, and dyspnea/breathlessness/ respiratory problems, 97

seizures, as side effect of opioids, 136

Selective Serotonin Reuptake Inhibitors (SSRIs), 73–74, 77

senna, 88

senna (Senokot), 127

senna tea, 86

senses, as ways of connecting to loved one, 54

Seroquel (quetiapine), 93, 94, 135

Serotonin-Norepinephrine Reuptake Inhibitors (SNRIs), 74, 77, 116

shame, of family members about dementia, 52, 53

shock, as reaction to diagnosis, 8

shortness of breath (dyspnea). see dyspnea (shortness of breath)

shouting, as nonverbal cue, 60

sight, as way of connecting to loved one, 55

silence
around issues of end-stage dementia, 9, 12
around process of death and dying, 8

silver sulphadiazine, 105

Sinequan (doxepin), 73, 130

skin breakdown
approaches/interventions for, 104–108, 131–135
causes of, 103–104
clinical presentation of, 102–103

skin care, 107, 130

sliding scale approach, to capacity determinations, 30

smell, as way of connecting to loved one, 54

smoking, as risk factor for dementia, 4

SNRIs (Serotonin-Norepinephrine Reuptake Inhibitors), 74, 77, 116, 125

social workers, 42, 63, 69

sodium phosphates, 84–85, 87

Solomon, S., 19

solumedrol, 95

somatic symptoms, 71

sorbital, 86

sores, pressure, 102–107

speech pathologists, 101

splinting, as non-pharmacologic adjuvant, 120, 124

SR (sustained release) preparations, 123

SSRIs (Selective Serotonin Reuptake Inhibitors), 73–74, 77

St. John's Wort, 75

starvation, 37

Stemetil (prochlorperazine), 90, 126

STERI/SOL mouthwash, 138

Steroid Equivalency Chart, 142

steroids, 95, 96, 99, 102, 124, 130, 138, 139, 142

stimulating agents, for constipation treatment, 85

stomatitis, as side effect of opioids, 138

stool softeners, 83

straws, cautions with, 98

subcutaneous hydration (hypodermocylsis), 109

subcutaneous injections, 141

substitute decision-maker (SDM), 26, 29, 30–31, 38, 39–40, 47, 63, 143

substitute judgment, 147

sucralfate, 100, 105, 138

suctioning, 97

suffering
artificial hydration/nutrition and, 38, 39
avoidance of, 46, 47
and ethical approach, 26
of family members, 56
hunger and, 37
medical advances and, 7, 13, 15
and pain treatment, 40, 111, 117
and palliative care approach, 9, 15, 18, 20, 32
patients' views on, 28, 35

support, importance of, for patients and caregivers, 21

suppositories, 86, 127

surgical fixation, as non-pharmacologic adjuvant, 120, 124

surrogate decision-maker, 147. *see also* substitute decision-maker (SDM)

sustained release (SR) preparations, 123

sweating, as nonverbal cue, 60

symptom assessment
difficulty of, 67
general guide for, 68, 117
instruments of, 72
reluctance to report symptoms, 68

symptom control/management, 48, 67–110, 121–141

symptoms
of anxiety, 75–77
of constipation, 81–88
of dehydration, 107–110
of depression, 71
of dysphagia/oral complications, 97–98
of dyspnea/breathlessness/respiratory problems, 94
of nausea/vomiting, 88–91
neuro-vegetative symptoms, 72
of pain, 110–111. *see also specific pains*
relief of, 39–40

of skin breakdown/chronic wounds, 102–103
somatic symptoms, 71
vegetative symptoms, 71
of weight loss/anorexia/cachexia, 77–81

T

tactile experiences, 54

Tantum (benzydamine HCl), 138

Tegretol (carbamazepine), 125

Tehchkoff™ catheter, 96

tenacious sputum, 95

TENS (Transcutaneous Electronic Nerve Stimulation), 70, 115, 120, 125

terminal airway secretions ("death rattle"), 140

terminal diseases, 11, 12

terminal restlessness, 77

tetracycline, 99

therapeutic touch, 76, 81, 94, 95, 117, 120

thoracentesis, 96, 140

thromboplastin, 105

titration, 69, 73, 74, 109, 115, 116, 117, 123, 130, 135

touch
massage. *see* massage therapy
role of, 48
therapeutic touch. *see* therapeutic touch
as way of connecting to loved one, 54

traditional Chinese medicine, 81

tramadol (Ultram), 113, 114, 115, 120, 121

tranquilizers, 5

transcendence, 54

Transcutaneous Electronic Nerve Stimulation (TENS), 70, 115, 120, 125 trazodone, 77

tricyclic antidepressants, 73, 82, 98, 99, 115, 116, 124

tube feeding, 17, 38, 42, 146. *see also* feeding tubes

U

ulcerations, as side effect of opioids, 138

ulcers, 100, 102

Ultram (tramadol), 113, 114, 115, 120, 121

ultrasound, as non-pharmacologic adjuvant, 120

United States, as melting pot, 45

V

Valium (diazepam), 128, 136

valproic acid, 125

vaporizer, 97, 110

vascular (multi-infarct) dementia, 4

vegetative symptoms, 71

ventilator, 146, 147

ventolin, 139

veracity, as ethical term, 147

verbal expression, patient's lack of, 58

Versed (midazolam), 97, 105, 128, 135, 136, 139

vestibular disturbances, and nausea/vomiting, 89, 90

visceral disturbances, and nausea/vomiting, 89

visual stimulation, value of, 55

voice
   of health care professionals, 56
   wet voice, 98

Volicer, L., 14

vomiting
   approaches/interventions for, 90

causes of, 89

clinical presentation of, 88

as side effect of opioids, 126

vulnerability, of patient, 147

W

wasting (cachexia)
   approaches/interventions for, 78–81
   causes of, 78
   clinical presentation of, 77–78

weight loss
   approaches/interventions for, 78–80
   causes of, 78
   clinical presentation of, 78

wet voice, 98

World Health Organization (WHO), 106, 113

wound healing, 107

wound procedures, cautions with, 106

written record, of patient's wishes and values, 63. *see also* advance directive

X

xylocaine, 138

Z

Zantac (H2 antagonists), 91, 100

Zyprexa (olanzapine), 79, 80, 90, 93, 94

Lightning Source UK Ltd.
Milton Keynes UK
UKOW040125041212

203122UK00001B/48/P